ROCKFORD PUBLIC LIBRARY

Rockford, Illinois

http://www.rpl.rockford.org

DEC 04 2002

DEMCO

Nature's Ritalin
for the Marathon Mind

Disclaimers

1. The names, identities, genders and descriptions of parents and children used in examples and case histories have been changed. Resemblance to anyone is purely coincidental.

2. Exercise is not a mental cure-all. Diagnosis and treatment of ADHD requires consultation with appropriate professionals. While exercise is an appropriate adjunct treatment, its use as a substitute for medication or therapy requires consultation with a physician, psychiatrist, or psychotherapist. A physical exam is essential before embarking on a new exercise regimen. Some forms of exercise require training by certified specialists.

Nature's Ritalin for the Marathon Mind

Nurturing your ADHD Child with Exercise

Stephen C. Putnam

Foreword by W. Mark Shipman, M.D.

Upper Access, Inc., Book Publishers
Hinesburg, VT
http://www.uppperaccess.com

Nature's Ritalin for the Marathon Mind: Nurturing your ADHD Child with Exercise is published by Upper Access Book Publishers, an imprint of Upper Access, Inc.

Upper Access, Inc.
85 Upper Access Road
PO Box 457
Hinesburg, VT 05461-0457

Web: *http://www.upperaccess.com*
E-Mail: *info@upperaccess.com*
Telephone for orders: 800/310-8320
Telephone for other business: 802/482-2988
Fax: 802/482-3125

ISBN: 0-942679-26-1
Library of Congress Control Number: 2001017887

Library of Congress Cataloging-in Publication Data

Nature's ritalin for the marathon mind : nurturing your ADHD child with exercise / by Steve Putnam ; foreword by Mark Shipman.
p.   cm.
Includes bibliographical references and index.
ISBN 0-942679-26-1 (trade paper : alk. paper)
1. Attention-deficit hyperactivity disorder–Exercise therapy. 2. Attention-deficit hyperactivity disorder–Alternative treatment. I. Putnam, Steve (Stephen C.), 1948-

RJ506.H9 N38   2001
618.92'8589062–dc21   2001017887
CIP

Printed in the United States of America on acid-free paper

Table of Contents

Acknowledgments

The idea that physical exercise promotes mental health is not new. Keepers of the flame—writers, researchers, educators, and parents—have managed to keep this idea alive over the years. Researchers and writers whose works have influenced this book are listed in the endnotes and bibliography.

I am also indebted to all of the parents who shared stories about the ways exercise helped their children cope with ADHD—with and without medication.

At risk of leaving someone out, I'm indebted to the following people who helped bring these ideas together from a number of different scientific and professional disciplines.

Eduardo Bustamante was the first to encourage me to write *Nature's Ritalin for the Marathon Mind.* He also warned me about the challenges of convincing parents and children that exercise does more than help build a strong body.

While Dr. Stuart Copans was serving as guest editor for *Reaching Today's Youth,* published by National Education Service, he and I wrote an article on exercise for ADHD children. Through Stuart, I learned that evolutionary psychology is taken seriously in the medical community. In a world that often limits our movement, exercise is a logical solution to mental needs with evolutionary roots.

Ronald E. Jones, director of the Attention Deficit Disorder Clinic in Washington State, and Gretchen May, a therapist in Massachusetts, were the first to introduce the idea that brief physical movement can have immediate effects.

Journals and magazines have introduced me to a number of researchers, practitioners, and educators who have witnessed the miracles of exercise.

Some of the authors of studies cited in this book include C. Bass,

Jill Allen, and W. Mark Shipman, all of whom spent time on the phone answering questions and adding insights that weren't included in their published studies.

Two educators, Jeanette Girard and Rick D'Elia, read an early draft of *Nature's Ritalin for the Marathon Mind.* Their comments made me aware of the time constraints of teachers in today's classrooms. If it weren't for them, I would still be working with a few naive assumptions about most public school settings.

The people at Concept II connected me with educators who answered survey questions that were used as a reality check—do physical education teachers see the same behavioral improvements that researchers see? Among the schools contacted was Ballenger Creek Middle School in Maryland, which has a physical education department that's more progressive than most. Classes meet five times a week and aerobic exercise is a requirement in every student's personal fitness plan. Its director, Carol Baker, took the survey a logical step further by passing a questionnaire around to academic teachers. Carolyn Frodyl, also an educator at Ballenger Creek, knew of real-world instances in which exercise has been successfully mixed into student routines.

Ian Harling, a former student and canoe-trip leader, and Mike Maunder, a former teacher at St. John's Anglican Boarding School in Canada, provided much of the background on that school.

I need to thank Steve Carlson, publisher and primary editor, for sharing the same vision, avoiding exaggeration, and keeping the message on track.

And thanks to my friend Cindy Lydiard, who doesn't need as much exercise as I need to maintain neurochemical levels necessary for continuous optimism. Her enthusiasm helped to carry this project through to completion.

Foreword
by W. Mark Shipman, M.D. *

The obvious is often a difficult sell. The relationship between tobacco and disease is a contemporary example. As long as 50 years ago, tobacco's partnership with lung cancer, emphysema, and heart disease was as apparent as the melanomas on our sun-tanned faces. Yet we chose to ignore the obvious in favor of the seductive advertising that made cigarettes seem sexy, stylish, and "in."

The fact that aerobic exercise promotes normalcy has also been an elusive reality for our society. Today, Americans cling to the dream that conveniences delivered by technology will lead us to Nirvana, even while our bodies atrophy and our brains become alarmed and depressed. We ignore the obvious truth that our central nervous systems evolved with physical activity, not a couch-potato lifestyle. We do so at our peril. As a nation, our weight is paralleling our wealth, and our shadow is widening along with our influence.

Back in 1978 at the San Diego Center for Children—where ADHD is the rule among children in treatment—an uncontrolled study found dramatic reduction in the use of medication by children who were engaged in a running program. However, amazingly, more

---

* Dr. Shipman is Director of the Institute for Developmental Research at the San Diego Center for Children, and Associate Clinical Professor of Psychiatry at the University of California Medical School at San Diego.

5

than 22 years later, aerobic exercise is still rarely included on any list of treatment options for ADHD.

A recent extensive study, funded by the National Institute of Mental Health, compared various treatment approaches for ADHD in combination and alone. Exercise was not even included for consideration!

Exercise just isn't taken seriously. We question anything so obvious and profound. "How could it be so easy?" It's like Plato's Cave. "Don't bother us with reality. We are busy discussing these shadows on the wall."

Most adults who work with ADHD children would probably agree that exercise is a good idea, just as most health-care professionals half a century ago probably agreed that smoking was harmful to health. Within the next half century, our society will undoubtedly warm up to the obvious and include exercise as a part of every ADHD treatment plan. But that will come too late to help today's children if we are slow in making the change. The benefits are attainable today, as this book makes clear.

Steve Putnam reviews and discusses in this volume the reasons for the paradox between the evidence and the practice regarding the application of aerobic exercise in ADHD management.

There may be some understandable reasons why we talk the talk but don't go for the walk. Certainly the chaos surrounding life with ADHD children works against any notion of encouraging more activity. We want them quieter, not more active. Medication often helps, so it's tempting to believe that is the whole solution and nothing else is needed. It is certainly easier to prescribe pills than to suggest and oversee exercise programs.

Steve Putnam has done a convincing job of building the case for including exercise in the treatment of children with ADHD. He takes a refreshingly comprehensive view of the subject and includes abundant and attractive practical advice. Especially important are the allowances for "different strokes for different folks." Everybody has different needs, and our needs change at different times in life.

For example, my own running efforts began at a time in my life when I was overweight and hypertensive. My dog was an Afghan hound who needed daily aerobic exercise to remain sane. He got me started, and together we ran hundreds of miles. I enjoyed it so much that I began entering marathons. My present pet is a much mellower Golden Retriever who is far better suited to my two-decade-older frame. My Afghan days are over.

Children vary greatly in their makeup, both physical and mental. The book strongly appeals to these variations, with practical advice for determining the optimal activities for any specific child. It also provides excellent advice on how to encourage children to take on an exercise program and stick with it.

The whole notion of a "mind-body connection" has always baffled me, since it seems clear that there really is no separateness in the first place—only a different view of the sameness. Steve clearly concurs. We think, therefore we are. We exercise, therefore we change. It's a simultaneously simple and intricate concept.

Overall, the use of exercise to help adults with anxiety and depression is much more widely substantiated in the literature than its use with ADHD. However, at a recent postgraduate education seminar I attended on that topic, exercise was missing from the recommendations. Nevertheless, during a question-and-answer period, attendees were polled on whether they believed exercise to be effective in the management of anxiety and depression. Eighty percent responded "Yes."

Dr. John Griest, chairman of the Department of Psychiatry at The University of Wisconsin and one of the earliest researchers on the relationship between aerobic exercise and emotions, shared his opinion with me that aerobic exercise is as effective as any other treatment for mild-to-moderate anxiety and depression. When asked his opinion about possible neurochemical mechanisms to explain this phenomenon, he suggested multiple possibilities, including norepine-phrine, serotonin, dopamine, and endorphins, as well as currently unknown "secondary messengers."

The exercise message seems to be an easier sell among seniors than among parents and caretakers of ADHD children. Exercise and an emphasis on fitness permeate programs for those in their "golden years." At age 71, during a TV interview, a friend was asked, "What do you see as the main benefit for you from running?" The answer was, "Problem solving. . . . No doubt about it. I can be struggling over some problem in my life, some puzzle that's hounding me. I go for a run, and 20 minutes into it, 'Bang!' I have the answer. I can depend on it."

In 1980, I ran the Avenue of the Giants Marathon through the Redwood Forest in northern California in the company of a fascinating man. Richard Bangler, M.D., was 80 years of age, and that day he set the world-record marathon time for octogenarians. For nearly four hours we ambled along together, and he told convincing tales from his life experience. He talked of how running had kept his mind sharp and his mental energy surging. Ten years later, I saw Dr. Bangler on a TV special about outstanding people in their 90s. He was still running.

Again and again, people discover and rediscover later in life how exercise can help them to overcome anxiety and focus their minds. How can it be any different for children who are anxious and unfocused?

I find this volume very exciting. It makes avoiding the obvious extremely difficult. It could have a major impact on our lives and the lives of our children. I hope we'll take heed.

It could well be that upon reading *Nature's Ritalin,* you may feel inspired to exercise along with the children you supervise. If so, go for it! As Kostrubala noted in *Running as Therapy,** if we think of psychotherapy as being like a garden, the psychotherapist (or the adult playing that role) is the gardener. Running is a tool that may change both the garden *and* the gardener.

Steve Putnam explores the complexities of the issues in this book. It's always dangerous to reduce important issues to a few simple words. But as a general guiding principle, I like the saying on the refrigerator magnet: "Move your butt. Your mind will follow."

---

*See Endnote #51

The Marathon Mind
and the Granola Effect

1

... And when we're not being tested—by the weather,
by predators, by other tribes—several million years of
evolution go unused . . . .
> —*Sebastion Junger* [1]

How did our ancestors survive without Ritalin®?* One answer to this question has long been apparent to a few educators and parents who understood the psychological value of exercise.

As recently as the 1970s and early '80s, when Ritalin was still making its debut, some doctors were referring "problem kids" to St. John's Anglican Boarding School, a Canadian private school that operated with the Outward Bound philosophy that hardship creates character. St. John's philosophy has evolved with the times, but, like many other private schools, it still operates on the belief that academic and career successes depend on exposure to sports and outdoor programs. Outdoor programs include canoeing, hiking, camping, snowshoeing, and dog-sledding. Sports include soccer, football, hockey, volleyball, basketball, and lacrosse. The programs develop confidence and leadership abilities, teach life skills such as the work ethic, and promote endurance and stress management.

In the 1970s, some of St. John's students began showing up with Ritalin. One teacher decided that the students who brought Ritalin for

---

* Ritalin is a trade name, registered by Novartis Pharmaceuticals Corp., for the drug methylphenidate.

their three-week canoe trips wouldn't need it. When you cover 30 miles a day by canoe, you don't need to take extra steps to calm anyone down, he noted. You actually need lots of activity. After a trip, the teacher often took parents aside to assure them that their children were fine without Ritalin.

The Marathon Mind

The term "Marathon Mind" might be a better label for ADHD, a condition with behaviors that often reflect a need for constant physical and mental movement.

Children with ADHD are often described as hyperactive, impulsive, and inattentive. They appear to be non-stop thinkers or scanners. Some live in a dream world, some thrive on novelty. While there seems to be a lack of control, there's usually plenty of momentum. When the momentum is lost, depression can result.

In many cases and many ways, the marathon mind's need for constant stimulation is normal and healthy. The term Attention Deficit Hyperactivity Disorder might make some children feel like victims who somehow lost in a genetic crap shoot. That description alone could conceivably contribute to depression.

While psychostimulant medication increases attention, it also reduces playfulness, another necessary component of childhood development. While this book will present evidence that suggests that the chemical benefits of exercise are at least comparable to the benefits of medication, it will also present some speculation from a leading neuroscientist, Jaak Panksepp, who believes that play is a mammalian birthright. Short-circuiting the brain's need for play may have undesirable consequences.[2]

One concern about the chemical stimulation provided by medication is that it is a form of repression that breeds conformity. Medication's saving grace lies in its ability to at least make the classroom more tolerable for some children who suffer with ADHD. At best, it can enhance academic functioning. Along with medication, or sometimes in place of medication, you can teach your child to make use of the best stimulation that the environment already offers. You can nurture your child's psychological development with simple exercise.

Drugs as the Treatment of Choice

Since the 1970s, attention-deficit disorder has become the fastest-growing diagnostic category for children. A group of health-care providers in New York State reported that almost 19 percent of all pediatric visits involved psycho-social problems in 1996—more than two and a half times as many psycho-social problem visits as there were in 1976.

The rate of increase was greatest for children between four and fifteen years of age, and drugs became the treatment of choice. In 1996, 78 percent of the children diagnosed with attention deficit/hyperactivity disorder (ADHD) were taking medication, two and a half times the 32 percent who were taking medication in 1979.[3]

At the incremental rate that ADHD has been diagnosed in the twentieth century, an estimated 15% of American children may be diagnosed with the disorder in the early 21st century.[2]

There is nothing particularly surprising about the rise of drugs as the treatment of choice for a condition that is becoming increasingly pervasive.

A truly effective effort to resolve psychological problems requires coordination among all those interested in a child's well-being.[3] Treatment is often frustrating and time-consuming. Pediatricians can't change the school system. Therapists can't change parents who don't spend enough time with their children at home. Parents can't change their children's peer groups. Most of the time, teachers can't take their students out for a run. Could it be that school districts, insurance companies, and stressed parents see medication as a quick fix for this complicated problem?

The Dangers of Simplistic, Extreme Positions

News media discussions ignore the diagnostic complexities of attention-deficit disorder and present a debate that pushes people into polarized positions based on personal beliefs rather than medical certainties. The impression is that one needs to either be "for" or "against" drugs. There is a tendency for those who support drugs to rule out other useful therapies, and for those who oppose drugs to latch onto anything else, regardless of whether it has been shown to work. Many act as if there are only two possible options—medicine or good old-fashioned willpower and responsibility.

This polarity is also reflected in recent class-action lawsuits that allege that Ritalin's manufacturer conspired with the American Psychiatric Association to invent the standards for ADHD diagnosis, using a broad variety of symptoms that could apply to any child. The nonprofit support group Children and Adults with Attention Deficit/ Hyperactivity Disorder (CHADD) has also become a target of this class-action suit.

Is the disorder real or imagined? Are psychostimulant meds effective or ineffective, safe or dangerous? No matter what we believe about ADHD and medication, polarized views won't help parents and teachers of children who have trouble functioning at home and at school.

There's too much at stake to choose one or the other based on our personal beliefs—either romantic ideas about natural remedies or blind faith in medicine. It really is more complicated than that. For starters, ADHD does not always have the same exact symptoms and causes.

Aside from diagnostic questions best left to qualified doctors and psychologists, and aside from the debate between those who believe that ADHD is a fictitious construct of the pharmaceutical community and those who believe that ADHD is medically credible, the behavioral, academic, and social problems remain. The efficacy of medication has been proven, to some degree, for children living in modern environments under conditions unprecedented in human history.

12

The causes of ADHD range from genetic inheritance to ingestion of lead. The condition varies from mild to severe, and in subtype from hypoactive to hyperactive. There may be co-morbidity—in other words, it may coexist with another category of learning disorders such as dyslexia. Symptoms of depression and other psychological conditions can mimic those of ADHD and vice versa. To complicate things even further, a child who is diagnosed as ADHD by one physician or psychologist might be diagnosed as normal by another. Both might describe him or her as highly creative, adventuresome, or personable. Since ADHD takes on so many symptomatic forms, any blanket statement about medication or any other treatment mode is likely to be inaccurate.

The Pros and Cons of Medication

There are a number of books and articles advancing the argument that medication is inherently bad. This is not one of them. Lab studies have proven in many cases the effectiveness of psychostimulant medications such as Ritalin, and real-world doctors and parents have seen these medications improve attention, impulse control, and mood.

It is also a fact of life—unfortunate but true—that financial realities often dictate treatment. If a psychological disorder has biological roots, insurance will more likely cover medication than extended psychiatry or other forms of therapy. When you consider the expense of psychotherapy or hiring a personal exercise coach, medication may be the most cost-effective option available.

On the other hand, some argue that Ritalin and other psychostimulant medications may stunt growth, cause rebound effects, increase blood pressure, and cause weight loss. Researchers report that the brain may become sensitized to Ritalin and similar drugs, and also might have long-term toxic effects on the brain.[4]

Drug therapy poses numerous potential risks. Some children forget—and some refuse—to take medication, especially those who are self-conscious about going to the school nurse's office for meds. Adolescents may experiment with drug cocktails, a mix of pills from more than one prescription. On occasion, the media report rare but extreme side effects such as heart damage. For parents, the decision on whether their children should take medication is a risk-management question. Do the risks of ADHD behavior outweigh the risk of medication?

Exercise as an Alternative

Many parents of ADHD children are looking for viable alternative therapies that can complement, and perhaps eliminate the need for, medication. No matter what position parents take on the medication issue, exercise provides an additional option. Based on the limited research that is available, it is effective with children who take medication as well as with those who don't.

The idea that exercise has psychological benefits has not gone unnoticed by government agencies and non-profit organizations that serve the interests of children. The Surgeon General's Report of 1996 finds that inactivity leads to a deterioration of mental health.[5]

According to Child's Right to Play (IPA/USA), an organization that advocates recess for children, physical movement often relieves attention-deficit symptoms. The group also suggests that Americans could learn from other countries, such as Japan, where long classroom sessions alternate with intense periods of outdoor play.[6]

As you will see later in this book, extreme forms of sensory deprivation, including immobility, can trigger attention-deficit symptoms in *anyone*. These symptoms include inattentiveness and hyperactivity.

Victims of Inactivity

Twenty-first-century technology makes many of us victims of inactivity. Most of us, including children, have far fewer physical chores than did past generations. We also have far more opportunities for leisure activities that make use of joysticks, mice, and remote-control devices rather than muscles. Given what we know about the effects of exercise on the brain and the consequences of lack of exercise, the staggering increase in ADHD should come as no surprise.

Most likely, genetic makeup predisposes some children to ADHD behavior. From an evolutionary biological point of view, some things that we consider diseases or disorders may have served as useful functions at the time that they evolved. If this is the case, at least *some* ADHD cases can probably be more accurately identified as a disorder of adaptation rather than a result of genetically caused brain abnormalities.[7] While sickle-cell anemia is an illness in the western world, it protected people from malaria in Africa, where it evolved.[8] Some ADHD diagnoses may be a result of genetic makeup *combined* with modern lifestyles that are made possible by a more comfortable environment.

Thousands of years of evolution have provided the best preparation for situations that require physical prowess and quick thinking, both attributes of a marathon mind. Out of necessity, many contemporary school and work environments suddenly discriminate against these attributes. In the past, environment and genetic makeup were less likely to conflict. The runner would be more likely to outrun a lion if he could outsmart him as well.

We often compartmentalize ideas of physical exercise and intellectual exercise. Many in our 21st century world constantly distinguish between athletic jocks and intellectual geeks, almost as separate categories of people. It's easy to forget that the mind and body function as one. As our species evolved, in all likelihood, intelligent runners out-survived counterparts who were only intelligent or only fast runners. And, as we now know, running (among other physical activities that influence blood flow and oxygen intake) also enhanced mental functioning.

In practice, the same children who respond most to psycho-stimulants seem to also respond most to exercise. Since all of us have a threshold at which inactivity affects us in a negative way, exercise is important for everybody's mental health.

Available research with ADHD children has often been informal, but there is enough lab and anecdotal evidence to make a convincing case for the benefits of exercise. More research might provide more clues for determining how much exercise is optimal, although it is clear that everyone is unique in that regard. Unfortunately, extensive new research is unlikely to happen until someone finds a way to make as much money promoting exercise as the drug companies make from their patents.

Exercise may not be a cure-all for ADHD. But the evidence is strong that treatment plans that *don't* include exercise are missing a vital factor in brain development and maintenance.

Caution Required when Reducing Medication

With these assumptions, parents should approach exercise therapy with a pragmatic attitude that asks, "How well does it work for my child?" Ideally, your child's doctor can monitor the effects of exercise using the same criteria used to monitor the effects of medication.

For parents who hope to discontinue medication for their children, drug withdrawal requires clinical supervision. In cases in which children are suffering from side effects of drugs, there may be a tendency to move too quickly. Stimulant meds, like other drugs, can produce withdrawal symptoms. Behavior can worsen temporarily. Mental symptoms ranging from fatigue to depression to suicidal tendencies are possible. In general, any withdrawal of medication should be gradual.[9]

Have we, as a society, substituted medication for the exercise that is no longer a routine part of life? That may be an overstatement. In practice, most would agree that the relative safety and convenience of modern life are, in an overall sense, highly welcome. However, restoring enjoyable forms ofexercise as a routine part of life helps many children to reduce or eliminate drugs and increase their overall quality of life.

How Much Exercise?

The belief that exercise helps children to "let off steam" is not precisely accurate, but does generally describe the way it triggers neurochemical change and decreases restlessness. At certain extremes, either too much exercise or too little may be perceived as abusive. Where do the boundaries lie, in either direction?

The question of how intense the exercise should be does not necessarily need to be answered with a rigid recipe or prescription. Some of the best personal or group exercise programs have been based on intuition rather than a prescribed dosage.

However, for parents who claim that their child exercises already and that it doesn't seem to help, an effort to codify the scheduling and intensity of the activities may be very useful. Intelligent scheduling can also guard against the other extreme. With exercise, more is not always better. And any regimen that is too rigid or intense is likely to fail if the child dislikes it.

Good old-fashioned age-appropriate fun makes a good base from which to start. A general understanding of the effects of different intensities and durations of exercise is useful but should be adapted to fit your child's age, personality, and schedule.

At one relative extreme, St. John's takes its students on long-distance canoe trips that last three or four weeks, depending on how long it takes to reach the destination. At a similarly high level is the father who helped his son train for Olympic-level ski racing and, as the training intensified, hired a part-time coach.

Compare these relatively intense activities with the child counselor who shoots a few hoops or goes for a short walk while discussing grades or classroom behavior with a student. Knowing the effects of exercise intensity can help you decide how to encourage your child. Instead of asking your young child to run faster, you can structure games to encourage running longer or more often.

A Variety of Benefits

While the mind-body connection gets lots of attention from holistic health practitioners, it's sometimes easy to forget about on a day-to-day basis. Yet some children intuitively value the ability of exercise to calm and focus their minds. One anecdote tells about a boy who suggests that a friend go bike riding to cope with her frustrations.[10] There may be less apparent, long-term benefits as well. Some studies have even linked exercise with reductions in teen pregnancy, an indirect benefit of decreased impulsivity for both girls and boys.[11]

Although exercise is not a miracle cure, it is a significant piece of the mental-health puzzle. Inactivity affects everyone, regardless of whether they're genetically predisposed to ADHD. In some cases, exercise might completely replace Ritalin or other psychostimulants. In other cases, it might complement medication or allow it to be reduced at some point. Parents of children who try exercise need to watch how it works and keep the doctor apprised of behavioral changes or mood swings.

For children who are functioning well already, exercise serves as a buffer against future stresses that life might bring. Parents who think that their child needs medication or exercise to alleviate severe psychological conditions should consult a psychologist or psychiatrist. If attention-deficit symptoms are severe or caused by stress or by a more severe psychological disorder, psychotherapy or medication may be needed. Let a qualified professional make these diagnostic determinations.

It is common knowledge that more boys than girls are diagnosed with ADHD. Most likely, girls are under-identified and under-served in diagnosis of risk for long-term academic, social, and emotional difficulties.[12] At this time, there has been no research that accounts for possible sex difference in the mental benefits of exercise for those with ADHD. Barring such findings from future research, we can assume that there are benefits for both.

The Granola Effect

Many in our society pretty much assume that exercise is good and that too much inactivity is bad. This type of belief is sometimes called the "granola effect." The fact that everybody sort of recognizes that there are benefits makes it hard to convince people that more study is necessary.[13] It also makes it hard to convince some people that exercise is a serious remedy for specific problems, on a par with medication. Drug companies have funded so much research that you could get caught in an avalanche of journal articles about Ritalin and other psychostimulants. You'd barely trip on a pile of articles about the effects of exercise on ADHD.

While hyperactivity is often a symptom of ADHD, movement satisfies the wanderer, hunter, farmer, and gatherer in all of us. Neither exercise nor psychostimulant medication can change a child's genetic makeup or boost his IQ. But parents who see behavioral and academic improvements and children who feel positive change will discover the emotional and behavioral freedom that movement can bring.

Using the label "marathon mind" is a logical extension of the idea that ADHD traits were more desirable in the past, when physical prowess was more necessary for survival. It's also logical that some children (and adults) need more physical or mental activity than others. If children are denied exercise, hyperactivity and other ADHD behaviors are more likely to result.

No matter what you believe about the diagnostic credibility of ADHD, the efficacy of psychostimulant medication, or the idea that traits favored by evolution clash with some modern environments, your child's social or academic problems are not imagined. Medication should be available for children who need it. But since physical activity serves as one of many regulatory mechanisms of mental functioning, it should also be available for children whose symptoms may be a partial result of restrictive environments.

Diagnosis and Evaluation of Needs

Doctors should not fear that they are venturing out of the mainstream by prescribing exercise, even though the idea may be new to some. They can evaluate the effects of exercise using the same criteria that they use for medication.

No matter what you believe about ADHD, if your child exhibits symptoms, don't jump to immediate conclusions. A great many medical problems have been mis-diagnosed as ADHD. These range from pinworms to reactions to medications and psychological responses to situational stresses such as parental divorce or a move to a new community.[14] A doctor's diagnosis, including a physical exam, is required for intelligent decisions about the need for exercise, medication, or psychotherapy.

Hardship, Exercise, and Optimal Stimulation 2

*The physical stress of labor has been largely elimi-
nated by the introduction of machines. As a result of
this development, man's "sense of movement" and
with it its natural relationship to his body have
deteriorated. Fundamental instincts and emotional
outlets that physical exercise, in its various forms,
had afforded in the past, are no longer available.*

—*Ernst Jokyl*[15]

We've already established that ADHD symptoms vary from person to person, so blanket statements about the disorder have limitations. In theory, however, someone with ADHD who exercises might have fewer symptoms than a person who doesn't exercise and hasn't been diagnosed with ADHD.

Some prisoners of war have reported that calisthenics combated the effects of isolation, an extreme form of sensory or stimulus deprivation.[16]

We will look in this chapter at some laboratory evidence that proves, in an exaggerated way, that exercise is one way to stimulate improved mental functioning for people who are experiencing sensory deprivation. Obviously, children with ADHD are not participants in sensory deprivation experiments. But they are usually more hyperactive in class or in routine, structured settings than they are at recess or other less-structured situations. Some theorists have suggested that hyperactive behavior may function to optimize stimulation—and attention.[17]

Compare the classroom setting with more "natural" settings that our genetics might have prepared us for. In the past, a potential supper (a live rabbit) or danger (a mountain lion) would probably stimulate a hunter more than multiplication tables would stimulate many of us today.

In the past, killing the rabbit or running away from the lion was a necessary physical act. It not only accomplished the immediate need to find food or escape danger but probably also modulated the person's neurochemistry, enabling him or her to think more quickly. Our mechanized farms and supermarkets make the process of acquiring food relatively free of stress and trouble, as long as we keep our children and ourselves functioning at optimal levels of arousal for academic and career survival.

If our modern environment is too comfortable, what can we do to create just the right amount of stimulation to keep functioning at peak levels? Since we devote so much energy, money, and medication trying to motivate our children, the effects of exercise on hyperactivity, impulsivity, and attention are worthy of consideration.

Proprioceptive feedback—sensory information that is produced within the body, often by movement—is one form of stimulation that we use, consciously or not, to adjust our arousal level as well as our sense of tranquility. Until the last century, exercise had always been an inherent component of life that took many traditional forms, ranging from tribal war to religious dances. Monks exercised to prepare for worship, Aboriginals walked the Australian bush on ritual journeys, and young Tohono O'odham Indian teenagers ran 40 miles through the Arizona desert as part of a coming-of-age ritual.

Today, some children squirm at their desks, tapping fingers or speaking out of turn with smart-aleck answers. Some sit and stare into space. They're trying to find a comfortable balance, believe it or not. They probably aren't succeeding, but you have to give them credit for trying. From their perspective, they're stuck in school—and this is the best they can do under these circumstances.

One possible antidote has been known for years. *Hypokinetic Disease,* a book about the consequences of inactivity, put it this way in 1961: "Parents and teachers as well as psychiatrists have seen children's moods change almost miraculously if they have sufficient opportunity for active play."[18]

In a great many ways in our modern society (at least in North America), we function with less exercise and greater physical comfort. Threats to our well-being are usually fewer and more remote than the immediate dangers posed by wild animals or war, so it's not surprising that overall activity has decreased.

The Down Side of Convenience

In the last 50 years, American children have come to spend more and more of their time at physically passive pursuits, such as watching TV (which provides vicarious danger), playing computer games, and just hanging around. Why not? There's less farm work. There's less open space and generally less opportunity to hunt for food. Most houses are warm in the winter.

There's nothing wrong with comfort. Most of us prefer the convenience of modern life to the relative hardship of the past. However, the fact that we are no longer *required* to routinely exercise can have a strong negative effect on our motivation to get the amount of exercise needed to function at an optimal level.

Mike Maunder, a former teacher at St. John's Anglican Boarding School, puts it this way. By car, we can travel 30 miles in a half hour. It usually takes all day to travel the same distance by canoe. While most of us don't rely on firewood for heat or cooking anymore, children still need to develop the character that they used to develop by chopping and splitting wood.

As times have gotten easier, we seem, as a society, to have become increasingly dependent upon Ritalin, Prozac, alcohol, cigarettes, and recreational pharmaceuticals. Is there a correlation between movement and mental health or is it just a coincidence?

This trend, of course, has been going on for quite a few years. As long ago as the beginning of World War II, research indicated that young merchant marine seamen died faster than the older ones when ships were torpedoed. This inability to hang on was attributed to the softer lifestyle in which the younger men had grown up.

In 1941, educator Kurt Hahn established the first Outward Bound program, in which students learned to overcome obstacles by sailing, hiking and canoeing. This program influenced some private school programs in North America, including St. John's Anglican Boarding School in Canada, which in the '70s had a reputation of being the toughest private school on the North American continent. In addition to its obvious physical demands, challenging exercise was shown to help build confidence, teamwork, and self esteem.

Of course, the concept has been expressed in different ways during different generations in various parts of the world. But it's not a new idea—it's just one that seems to need a revival in this period of history. Decreased stimulation that results from inactivity lowers our arousal level. Intentionally or not, outward-bound-type programs and boot-camp levels of training have provided a way to counteract some of the dysfunctions that might result from inactivity. They encourage functioning at an optimal level of performance.

The key word is "optimal." It is possible to get too much of a good thing. Even for well-trained athletes or soldiers, extreme over-exercise can lower glucose levels and cause fatigue-related symptoms— emotionality, mood disturbance, susceptibility to distractions, sleep problems, and appetite changes.[19]

Laboratory Evidence

Despite numerous examples, healthy skepticism could make you want to see more direct proof of a relationship between inactivity and impaired mental functioning. In the lab, severe sensory deprivation triggers symptoms similar to those of attention-deficit disorder. Immobility is a contributing cause, and exercise is a proven antidote.

Researchers sometimes use flotation tanks to study the effects of sensory deprivation. The tanks are large tubs filled with warm salt water for increased buoyancy. A cover eliminates visual input. White noise eliminates sound.

Such experiments have consistently shown that as your sensory input decreases, your mental ability deteriorates. You will have disorganized thoughts and decreased intellectual ability, and you will become inattentive. Eventually, you might begin to hallucinate. Even if you return to a more normal environment, electroencephalograph (EEG) irregularities will persist for three or four hours. Other monotonous sensory environments have caused disorganized brain functions similar to those caused by drugs or brain abnormalities.[20]

Now, suppose that the nature of the experiment is changed slightly. You spend a week in a flotation tank in an almost stimulus-free environment. However, this time, whenever your mental functioning seriously deteriorates, you're allowed to jump out of the tub and do calisthenics. At this point, you stop hallucinating. Your attention span and ability to concentrate improve.

Brief exercise counteracts the effects of isolation. Mental skills—including numerical and abstract reasoning, math problem solving, memory, and dexterity—improve.[16]

At the opposite extreme, too much stimulation makes life too stressful for optimal performance. If you've had a rough day at the office and you feel over-stimulated, a mental whiteout for an hour or two would be relaxing. You could relax in the same flotation tanks used to study the effects of sensory deprivation, as long as you don't immerse yourself for too long. Of course, an exercise break can help in this situation too.

Some children seem to do well academically without exercising. You could argue that this suggests that movement isn't necessary for optimal mental performance. However, the experimental results consistently show that inactivity impacts mental performance and that exercise helps restore optimal functioning.

If some of the achievers aren't exercising, what keeps them going? Are they using other sensory inputs such as TV to function on an optimal level? Since each of us has a different makeup, walking from class to class might be enough movement for some. We need to ask how much and what kind of exercise helps each of us function at peak mental levels. Some people need more than others. Children who are diagnosed with ADHD seem to need more physical movement than do other children.

Different Means of Arousal

A child's genetic makeup and environment help determine the amount of stimulation that is optimal for that child. The stimulation can take any of a number of different forms. The main ones are drugs, exposure to sensory stimuli, and exercise.

Some of us are prone to using chemical fixes, prescribed or not. We can drink coffee to wake up, smoke cigarettes to ponder problems, and calm down with a glass of wine. Some teenagers try smoking to project a rebellious or hip image and ultimately discover a new way to calm themselves. Obviously, nicotine is a terrible choice, with a huge cost in health, but there is little doubt that part of its allure is its ability, for some, to help calm the emotions and focus the mind. While Ritalin is a much better alternative, teens are often self-conscious about taking medication.

Meanwhile, we are constantly seeking different stimuli to promote mental equilibrium. Sights, sounds, odors, touch, and thought all provide stimulation. Cartoons, rock 'n roll, watching sport events, novels, or a search for a cure for the common cold can entertain our senses, more or less. Exercise is only one of many sources of stimulation.

In all likelihood, prime-time TV will arouse the average child more than a historical factoid from 1792 would. A sixteen-year-old may be able to improve concentration by reading *Hot Rod* instead of a history assignment. Unfortunately, the concentration may diminish again when it comes time to memorize geometry axioms.

The fact that life consists of more than just car magazines and rock 'n roll makes drugs and/or exercise more necessary. Longer-term educational and social goals require self-discipline that is difficult or impossible to achieve if the brain is in a low state of arousal. Great teachers and brilliant parents will help to make learning and growing experiences fun, but even they can't communicate necessary information to a child whose brain is in a state of chemical imbalance.

Because we have six senses, there are at least six basic ways to stimulate our minds. An ideal mix would employ all of the senses. Unfortunately, there is no perfect definition of what is ideal.

Both exercise and psychostimulants can increase our arousal levels to deal with everyday realities that are, in and of themselves, not particularly exciting. Reading a car magazine solves the excitement problem but doesn't solve the geometry problem. Since exercise is a missing component in the lives of many children, it provides a good place to start.

Not only does exercise enhance mental functioning, it can also serve as a vehicle for psychological development by teaching children how to overcome obstacles, train with peers or family members, and achieve personal goals. As with medication, exercise doesn't eliminate the need for other developmental necessities such as social contact, discipline, or intellectual stimulation.

From a parent's or teacher's point of view, alertness and academic performance are obvious goals. You also want your child to be more responsive or receptive to available social, academic, and family reward systems.

A child who is functioning at a peak level is calm, attentive, and more responsive because he doesn't have to generate unnecessary commotion to bring himself to an optimal level. A child who is calmer and less impulsive than usual is likely to have improved executive functions, and the ability to make better choices by considering probable payoffs for different options. The child might tackle the math homework sooner and read car magazines later, for instance. But the benefits should not just be described strictly in terms of academics; they are also important to social skills, street smarts, and every other attribute of a successful human being.

Runner's High

The paradoxical effects of exercise are similar to those of psychostimulant medications such as Ritalin. Both treatments can help a child become calmer and more alert. Although there may be some initial resistance to exercise, once a routine is established the motivation can build on itself.

To a child, avoiding distant prospects of heart disease or improving school grades may seem like nebulous rewards. However, exercise can become a behavior that rewards itself. Despite the many long-term benefits, most runners go for more immediate relaxation rather than longer lives or improved academics.

Runners use the term "runner's high" to describe feelings that might include elation, pain relief, and hyperfocus. Some of these runners are supporting a habit. Withdrawal can be painful. But exercise has far more potential as a positive addiction than as a negative one. The addictive potential, at its best, can be a powerful reward system for healthful activity.[21]

Both smokers and joggers are seeking mental equilibrium. Impulsive people with low arousal levels are more predisposed to try cigarettes or other recreational pharmaceuticals. Many of these same people might be predisposed to running, rowing, biking, or swimming since the neurochemical effects may impact them more than the average person.

Side Benefits

As noted above, it's highly possible that one of the appeals of nicotine is a decrease in hyperactivity. One behavior can substitute for another. Substance-abuse counselors have used exercise to help addicted people build a bridge from a negative addiction to a more positive one. Instead of relying on self-discipline to break their habits, some ex-smokers exercise.

You may be able to introduce your child to an alternative relaxation method before he or she decides to experiment with other methods of altering consciousness. One author, who links exercise with self-esteem, also suggests that teenagers who exercise are less inclined to try tobacco or other recreational drugs.[22]

At the risk of stating the obvious, many forms of exercise have other rewards as well. Most kids aspire to do well in sports. Being a member of a school or neighborhood sports team can be a source of pride and social triumph. Competence at informal sports, such as shooting baskets in the park, playing badminton in the back yard, or skating in the neighborhood rink can also be self-rewarding in terms of self-esteem and a means of gaining friends. A child inclined toward active sports may be able to use exercise exclusively to cope with symptoms of ADHD.

If your child is not naturally so inclined, a little nudging in that direction may be helpful. Putting up a basketball hoop against the garage if you have one, or giving the child a tennis racket instead of a video game for a birthday present, or buying a baseball glove for yourself in order to play catch and discuss baseball strategies may plant some positive seeds.

But some caution is required. If you don't recognize your child's predisposition to certain individual or group sports, you run the risk of pushing your child too hard in a specific direction. There can be backlash, and even an aversion to sports. We'll get more into that issue later in the book but it seems worth a brief mention here.

The important issue is exercise. If desire for athletic prowess is a motivation for exercise, then that's good. But it's important to understand that, even for those who have no aspiration to athletic achievements, exercise itself has substantial rewards. Ironically, some who don't think that they are competitive after trying group sports are surprised by their competitiveness in individual sports.

Maintaining Perspective

The psychology of exercise is a key element in the psychology of reward. The neurochemical changes that cause mood elevation also help children tune in and become more responsive to their environment. This is important, especially when sitting in a classroom or participating in other activities that require self-discipline. Psychostimulants such as Ritalin and exercise both provide similar neuro-chemical benefits for your child.

There may well be other sources of help. Psychotherapy, meditation, and special diets all have their advocates. Some believe that children just need to be told to take control themselves and exert some self-discipline. Other parents rely on threats like "Do your homework now, or else!" Or you may join millions of other parents in the decision that your child's problems are best solved with drugs.

The focus of this book is on exercise, because it has the potential to provide a huge amount of help to huge numbers of children. If it doesn't overcome your child's problems by itself, it should at least help, and complement other forms of treatment.

Out of necessity, educational, medical, and therapeutic practitioners tend to use the ADHD label to describe your child. At home and at school, it might be more helpful for your child to use the more positive label *marathon mind*. ADHD or not—victim or not—your child has to develop academically and socially. Identifying weaknesses and developing ways to cope are important steps. Fixating on a label can make your child feel like a victim or can isolate him or her from peers.

If for any reason you doubt that movement and exercise belong on the same page with attention deficit and hyperactivity, try a simple sensory deprivation experiment. See what happens:

- Wear a blindfold and ear protectors and lie on a mattress in a room that's not too hot or cold. (Make sure that you're not so tired that you sleep). Try not to move, sing, talk, etc. How long is this comfortable?

- Sit in a chair without moving, reading, talking, watching TV, or listening to music. What happens?

- After going through a period of sensory deprivation, try some exercises. Does the activity seem to speed up your return to feeling normal?

The Neurochemistry
of Optimal Stimulation

3

*"Exercise is yet another way that we can affect the
level and functioning of the neurotransmitter in the
brain. Exercise acutely causes the release of dopamine and serotonin. Chronic aerobic exercise leads to
an increase in the enzymes that make dopamine, so
exercise is not just a body issue, it's a brain trainer."*
—*John Ratey, co-author, Driven to Distraction*[23]

S o far, you have read about the possible effects of sensory
input on mental performance. Sensory input or "stress" can
mean anything from sound to sight to intellectual or emotional experience. It can mean the physical stress of exercise or
chemical stress of psychostimulant medication. How does medication, the favored treatment for ADHD, help to fulfill the need for
optimal stimulation? How does its alternative, exercise, fit?

A number of explanations might provide a rationale for the
effects of exercise on ADHD symptoms. First, we will look at a view
that encompasses the idea of play—as well as exercise. As noted
earlier, Dr. Jaak Panksepp believes that an understanding of circuits
that are built into the brain that promote play might help us understand ADHD. As already mentioned, psychostimulants reduce a
child's inclination to play.

Most likely, a child's play facilitates learning along with the
development of physical skills. It teaches certain social skills, ranging
from cooperation to parenting skills to the graceful acceptance of

defeat. In peaceful societies, sports might possibly provide a healthy substitute for aggression.[24]

According to Panksepp, "Without adequate daily outlets for such youthful energies, playful impulses will undoubtedly tend to intrude increasingly into regular classroom activities.[2] Panksepp advocates "Rough and Tumble play"—rough-housing. He notes that both inadequate and excessive levels of the neurochemical dopamine reduce play behavior, suggesting that we need normal dopamine levels to play.[24] In a later chapter of this book, we'll explore ways to determine how much rough-housing is appropriate.

Science has not yet come up with a truly comprehensive explanation of ADHD and how it is affected by medication or exercise. The neurochemicals that are affected by exercise include serotonin and dopamine, as well as the endorphin that is often associated with the "runner's high." Out of necessity, researchers study only bits and pieces of our neurochemistry at a time. To show that there is a relationship between hyperactivity, learning, and exercise, this chapter covers a few experiments that examine the effects of mostly one neurochemical, dopamine.

We have already seen the relationship between optimal stimulation and optimal mental functioning. Neurochemical changes accompany these psychological changes. For instance, dopamine levels increase or decrease, depending on medication intake, sensory stimulation, or exercise intensity.

Either exercise or medication relieves the well-known ADHD symptoms—inattention, hyperactivity, and impulsivity—while at the same time exerting an effect on our perception of reward.

Reward and Punishment

Parents and teachers often report that inattentive children will pay attention to tasks that excite them. When all is said and done, we either need to make tasks more exciting, or else we need to boost motivation with a psychostimulant drug or exercise.

Parents who use reward and punishment to control their child's behavior should understand that brain chemistry influences the success of any external reward system. The increased vigilance that we associate with medication may be an indirect result of the medication's effect on the brain's reward systems. We pay attention if we're excited enough to think that something is rewarding. Most likely, psychostimulants and exercise influence brain chemistry in ways that induce not only calming effects, but perceptual and motivational effects as well.

Generally, we think of reward as payment for certain behaviors. Teachers and behavioral psychologists who were educated in the '60s and '70s stress the importance of using tangible rewards and incentives to teach students and clients new behaviors. Thinking about reward in terms of the pleasure principle allows us to take a broader view. Some of the strongest rewards are produced internally. Even thinking about money we have not yet received can be rewarding. Real-life rewards often involve delay. Short-term neurochemical rewards are strong enough to keep us going in the meantime. In the real world, no one stands around passing out candy when we do good things and no one takes away recess when we do something they don't like.

How can there be internal rewards that are totally unrelated to the traditional rewards like food pellets for animals or candy for children? You can hook electrodes to certain points on a rat's brain and teach the rat to press a bar.[25] In return for electrical stimulation, the rat will press the bar for the rest of its life. In fact, it will give up sex and almost starve to death—just to keep its brain tickled.

The Role of Dopamine

Obviously, the external electrical source that controls the rat's mental functioning is artificial. Keep in mind that dopamine is probably one of the neurotransmitters that is providing a path for these electrons to move from neuron to neuron. There is no life-

33

sustaining reward in pure electrical stimulation, but a mental process, such as euphoria, will encourage the behavior that produces it.

What happens when you adjust the levels of neurochemicals that affect hyperactivity, attention, and learning? If you decrease the availability of the neurotransmitter dopamine, mental performance deteriorates—just as it deteriorates in prolonged sensory-deprivation experiments. The only difference this time is that you are directly changing brain chemistry rather than sensory or environmental input.

To test this, you can inject one five-day-old rat with a saline solution and inject another young rat with a dopamine blocker. Life will go on for both rats. Sensory input remains the same for both rats, but the one with low dopamine has decreased mental performance.

The saline-injected rat develops as a normal pup would. He is the usual busy young rat as he walks, runs, rears up on his hind legs, gnaws, eats, defecates, sniffs, grooms, scratches, licks, and washes himself. Most likely, these activities help young rats develop into psychologically mature rats.

Meanwhile, the rat that was injected with dopamine inhibitor is even busier. He does everything that the normal rat does, but he does everything much more often. "Hyperactive" seems like an appropriate way to describe him.

There are also long-term effects. In 28 days, the low-dopamine rat has outgrown his hyperactivity and, from all outward appearances, he seems normal. He is not, as you might have expected, a class clown. He takes school quite seriously.

The final test for the rats, before they can graduate, roughly resembles that of the gladiator in the short story *The Lady or the Tiger.* In the story, the gladiator has a choice between opening two doors. A beautiful lady waits behind one of the doors, and a hungry tiger waits behind the other. Similarly, the rats are given two doors to choose from.

Unlike the gladiator, each rat can take as many turns as he needs to pass the test. He stands on an electric shock grid, facing two doors on the other side of a 12-inch chasm. If he hesitates, he gets shocked. If he jumps across to the right door, it opens and he lands on a platform, safe. If he jumps across to the wrong door, it doesn't open and he falls into a net. Each rat graduates after choosing the correct door five times in a row.

Although the two rats appear similar, it takes more than twice as long for the dopamine-depleted rat to graduate. It's twice as hard and requires twice as many tries for this rat to make the choice that will lead to comfort and avoid the disturbance of falling into the net. After graduation, an analysis of the rats' brains shows that the dopamine concentration is still, indeed, 40 percent lower in the dopamine-depleted rat. This establishes that dopamine, in the right amount, helps a young rat to control its activity and to graduate from a laboratory experiment sooner.[26]

There is one obvious caveat to these experiments. Normality implies an optimal amount of dopamine, and in measuring performance we assume that a peak level is best. Who knows? Maybe, for the low-dopamine rat, the increased activity satisfies a healthy need for movement. Maybe the activity increase is a more appropriate response to the plexiglass that surrounds him. To a point, the dopamine-depleted rat worked a lot harder than a rat with a normal amount of dopamine. Maybe he needed more excitement. With people at least, this diversity isn't always inherently bad news, especially for societies that need soldiers, police, firefighters, emergency-room doctors, and race-car mechanics. Fortunately, not all brains are created equal. But they should all have equal opportunities to strive for equilibrium.

Psychostimulants and Dopamine

In general—depending on the dosage, situation, and person—psychostimulants can affect mood. When properly prescribed, they can often increase focus or reduce hyperactivity. In animal experiments, the same drugs act differently depending on an animal's genetic makeup. Experiments that measure effects of dopamine concentration in rats show that it affects hyperactivity and learning, and also affects perception of reward.[27] Most likely, increased dopamine levels are rewarding in and of themselves.

The paradoxical effect of amphetamine has been known for many years. In humans, psychostimulants increase available dopamine and reduce hyperactivity.[28] Your child can wake up and take a tab of Ritalin or one of the other psychostimulants with a glass of water to wash it down. The effects of most medications last for three or four hours. Jane may pay attention at school now. Johnny may not make as many smart-aleck remarks during class. Charlie might not fight as much.

One disadvantage of psychostimulants, which causes some psychiatrists to urge caution in their use, is that they have a "shotgun" effect on the brain, stimulating neurochemical production not just in areas where it's needed, but also where it's not needed. The optimal dosage for reducing hyperactivity might not be the optimal dosage for completing academic tasks.[29] A dose that maximizes performance in one academic area might not be the best dose for another. You could enhance a child's attentiveness *and* increase his anxiety at the same time, for example.

Equilibrium is never perfect and always involves compromise. But a good argument can be made that exercise, by invoking the body's natural processes, has a good chance of achieving more optimal effects than prescribed medication in a great many cases.

Getting High from Running or Drugs

Aside from optimizing our mental functioning, an even more immediate and attractive goal of exercise—or of prescribed or illicit medications—may be the resulting "high" or mood enhancement that often occurs.

Opium, a derivative of the poppy plant, has been available as a euphoric drug and pain killer for more than 4,000 years. One neurotransmitter that is linked to aerobic exercise has been called an *endorphin,* a pain-killing opiate that's produced within the brain. Popularization of the runner's high a few years ago made *endorphin* a household word. Many of the activities that people pursue for pleasure—such as sex, drug and alcohol use, and even eating—might trigger opiate-like reactions in the brain.[30] The endorphins produced by exercise seem to have the dual role of reducing pain and of providing an instant reward for a healthful level of activity.[30, 31]

The neurochemical changes that go with pleasure are complex and can't be explained with absolute certainty. Deserving or not, the runner's high and endorphins are treated in almost myth-like proportions. If you're a marathon runner, a self-produced pain killer is good, especially during the last part of the race when you need all of the pain killers you can get to make it to the finish line.

No matter what we're doing, we're constantly trying to fine-tune our brains to avoid pain, and, better yet, seek pleasure. Many of us spend the week working for comfort and security and spend the weekend trying to escape our ordered lives at night clubs, casinos, hikes, or canoe races. Excitement is rewarding. Reward is exciting. Pain killers, ranging from opium to the runner's high, can feel good even when we're not in pain.

Science or Spirituality?

You could suggest that a good run is like meditating, that repetitive movement is just like saying a mantra. Maybe the positive effects are religious or spiritual, or maybe the connection between exercise and an altered state of consciousness is just a coincidence. This book is not the best forum for discussion of theological issues. No particular set of beliefs is needed to augment the clear scientific evidence.

Compare active mice with littermates that had cages that were too small for any activity. The active mice lived in plexiglass health clubs with running wheels, ladders, and tunnels. They swam daily, learned to walk a tight rope, and climbed poles. In 17 days, the active mice had brains that weighed three percent more than the brains of their confined littermates.[32]

We can't draw conclusions about the spiritual aspects of exercise for mice, but there is a definite connection between what the body does for activity and how it develops. And exercise has immediate effects on neurochemistry. Mice who run for half an hour or swim for an hour metabolize greater amounts of dopamine than less-active littermates who stay in their cages, a finding that suggests that activity increases dopamine metabolism. [33]

You have already seen how blockers can reduce dopamine. While these conditions were obviously artificial, there are two ways that dopamine metabolism can be inhibited naturally. It's possible that some people are genetically predisposed to having brain chemistry that needs more dopamine than others. These same people are more likely to have symptoms that are commonly associated with ADHD.

The second natural dopamine blocker threatens all of us. Exercise avoidance, or physical rest, is brought to you by cars, power tools, computers, and television. If you feel drowsy when you get out of bed and notice that moving around wakes you up, you've identified the effects of rest and movement on your mood and level of alertness. You might notice that you wake up faster with activity on weekdays than you do on Sundays when you might not have to move as fast.

In the previous chapter, exercise compensated for sensory deficits and accompanying mental dysfunctions, including distractibility. When senses were deprived, psychological performance dropped off. If experimental participants exercise, psychological functions tend to normalize. Exercise is one of a number of ways to trigger this neuro-chemical process. In this chapter, we have seen how decreases in dopamine concentration inhibit mental functioning. We have also seen how dopamine concentration increases with exercise.

Other Possible Dopamine Stimulants

Again, both medication and exercise stimulate dopamine metabolism. Are there other conditions that do the same thing? What about stress that doesn't involve movement? A mouse that is immersed in cold water, shocked, or caged with a rat that's large enough to pose a threat will produce a greater amount of brain dopamine, even though it hasn't been moving.[33]

The dopamine metabolism that accompanies stress or excitement may explain the human attraction to extreme sports and may provide a more accurate description of what is happening when so-called adrenaline junkies describe the rush that accompanies excitement. When humans expose themselves to sports that involve danger, is it possible that they are dopamine-deficient and need to self-medicate with stress?

If exercise and stress trigger dopamine production, they should affect our perception of reward. Mood elevation is rewarding in itself, but these changes might also make a child more receptive to other rewarding opportunities—possibly ones that are available in the classroom.

Human Tests

Does exercise affect levels of dopamine in people like it does in animal experiments? We wouln't sacrifice humans as we do rats for neurochemical analysis, so scientists need other ways to analyze brain dopamine. Rather than give their lives to science, humans give vials of urine.

Dopamine serves its purpose connecting neurons so they can pass their electro-chemical messages, then breaks down into homovanillic acid, a by-product that passes in the urine. Urine or cerebrospinal fluid specimens provide a convenient way to reveal metabolic changes in the brain. Depressed people and hyperactive people, for instance, have less homovanillic acid in their urine, proof that they have a lower concentration of brain dopamine than most people.

The levels can be changed by activities alone, proving once again the strength of the mind-body connection. In one experiment, depressed patients ran in corridors, played ping pong, tennis, and pool. They also danced, sang, told jokes, did light calisthenics, drew murals, and disrupted people who weren't part of the experiment. Manic activity, or activity in itself, increased metabolism of three neurotransmitters, especially dopamine. The volunteers also reported mood elevation.[34]

To treat dopamine as if it is more important than any of the other neurotransmitter is, of course, simplistic. In reality, normal brain function is a result of neurotransmitters working in harmony with each other. And nothing proves that increased endorphin or dopamine levels cause mood elevation in rats or mice. We can only guess, because they don't know how to tell us. The animal research does suggest that exercise alters brain chemistry. If you've taken a hike or walked in the park recently, you probably didn't think of it that way, but the functional relationship between exercise and dopamine production is similar for animals and humans.

The Placebo Effect

One reason animal experimentation is so important is that humans are influenced by placebo effects. Do runners report highs because they're expected to? Or maybe they want their friends to know that they wouldn't waste time running unless there is something good about it.

Luckily, experimental rats don't know what the experimenter wants to see. Even if they did, why would they cooperate? A mind that is unaware of the researcher's motivation is an honest mind. If a rat quickly learns which door to choose and its brain contains more dopamine, or if a rat's mind has more dopamine after a swim, the results are probably reliable. With human tests, the results can always be questioned because of the complexities of the human mind and psychodynamics between experimenter and subject.

Yet the findings from human tests and personal experiences are convincing. To a point at least, we have some control over our ability to function at optimal levels. We can regulate our neurochemistry by exercising to increase dopamine levels.

If decreased amounts of dopamine reduce motivation and increase the time required for learning, then we can assume that, to a point, increasing available dopamine has the opposite effect. After exercising, depressed patients are less depressed and hyperactive children are calmer and more receptive to participating in learning tasks.

Paradoxically, activity calms the over-active mind, yet it can help motivate inactive ones.

Obviously, our needs vary, depending on our natural predispositions. The greatest benefits may be for those with a marathon mind.

Because exercise can elevate mood, it can be a self-perpetuating activity. Some athletes develop a positive addiction to the point that you can't stop them from exercising.

The potential of exercise can't be overestimated. Evidence suggests that our ability to master new information and remember old information is improved by biological changes in the brain brought on by physical activity. Practicing and learning complex movements causes the brain to grow more connections between neurons. Exercise that forces us to improve balance and coordination may not only help overcome clumsiness, but also reduce shyness.[35]

As we have seen, exercise causes neurochemical change. Recent animal research also suggests that running increases the production of neurons in a part of the brain that's responsible for memory and learning—in mice, running doubles the number of newborn brain cells that survive in this area. It also reduces the time required to learn certain tasks, and also enhances memory by strengthening synapse connections between cells.[36]

Dr. John Ratey believes that "Voluntary aerobic exercise is better than any other thing we can do . . . to have our daily dose of stem cells turn into live and vibrant new nerve cells. . . ."

If You're Not Yet Convinced . . ..

Here are some things to try, and/or to think about:

● On a day off from work, wake up and skip your coffee. How is your mood? Go for a half-hour walk. Has your mood improved or remained the same?

● After work, go for a half-hour walk (or jog) to see if there are any noticeable changes in your mood or behavior. Even if you already have a job that includes physical effort, the aerobic nature of walking may have some effect. If you're a parent, invite your child to accompany you.

• If you are not in condition to try intense exercise, ask an endurance athlete about exercise addiction. If exercise is the equivalent of hard labor, how can it be addictive?

Real-World Exercise and Optimal Stimulation

4

> *Daily exercise—briskly walking a few miles, for example—increases blood flow to the brain, or somehow otherwise alters body chemistry in a way that increases focusing ability for Hunters. . . . The daily run after the prey may well be a stimulant, or cause the release of hormones or neurotransmitters necessary for a Hunter's brain to work more smoothly.*
>
> —Thom Hartmann, *Attention Deficit Disorder: A Different Perception*[37]

As we have already noted, too much rest in a flotation tank makes people daydream and hallucinate. Dopamine blockers transform normal rats into hyperactive, slow learners. Theoretically at least, teaching a rat to swim might help it compensate for some of its mental deficits. In this chapter, we'll look at some of the studies and anecdotal evidence that confirm the positive, direct effects of exercise on children with ADHD.

The successful outcomes described here don't mean that you should make your own diagnosis and self-prescribe exercise to the exclusion of other treatments. A professional evaluation can allow other needed interventions as well. But the evidence is clear that aerobic exercise can often have at least the same benefits as medication in overcoming problems related to behavior and attention. It can also serve as a vehicle for social and psychological development, helping children to learn to overcome obstacles, to attain goals, and to participate in teamwork.

We'll also discuss the element of excitement, which, although the conclusions are somewhat speculative, seems to help motivate exercise and make behavioral outcomes more successful.

Remember how dopamine-limited, hyperactive rat pups were always busy as they walked, ran, stood on their hind legs, and scratched themselves more often than their normal brothers and sisters? Hyperactive kids are a little more complex. They irritate and worry teachers and parents. Some might be anxious or depressed. In classrooms, they're usually the ones who hit or bother classmates, call names, throw things, yell, talk out of turn, move around, or sit in their chairs the wrong way. They're less likely to cooperate, or take part in class, or follow instructions. They're more likely to have temper tantrums. Instead of doing their assignments, they'll daydream or doodle.

As we have already seen, stimulation can help regulate our emotions and behavioral patterns. Attempts to produce some of this needed sensory input might be as subtle as drumming fingers or as blatant as starting an argument. These efforts to focus are counterproductive. What can you do if you're the teacher? When these children are punished for making what may be paradoxical attempts to slow down and pay attention, the punishment often involves "time out" periods that restrict movement even more.

So far, research on the psychological effects of exercise has remained relatively obscure. Most of the teachers, doctors, and psychologists who have conducted field research on this subject are runners themselves. Most likely, they had experienced sufficiently beneficial effects from running themselves to make them want to see whether running might help children, especially those who were impulsive and hyperactive.

The following studies have similar, successful outcomes. They have enough differences in study design to provide results that suggest a wide range of exercise strategies that you and your child might try.

Classroom Studies

In two classroom studies, teachers compared student behavior on days that the children ran before class with days that they didn't. Running improved attention span and impulse control, and decreased the number of classroom disruptions by a half—for two to four hours.[38,39] One of these teachers, Jill Allen, continued to do morning runs with every one of her classes over ten years until her students were assigned to regular classrooms. While mixing special-needs students with mainstream students has its benefits, some of these students may have become victims of exercise deprivation. Unless students join track or cross-country teams, it's unlikely that anyone in the school system will have time to take them jogging.

Another researcher used a variety of clinical tests, along with evaluations by parents and teachers, to see how after-school exercise would affect hyperactive boys who weren't taking medication. This researcher screened out subjects with other disorders that might confuse the results, and also used more strict definitions of hyperactivity. The boys ran after school, three times a week, and the researcher monitored the intensity of the 15-minute runs. Teachers reported less hyperactivity at school on the following days.

Overall, light aerobic exercise seemed comparable to a low dosage of stimulant drugs. The boys had substantial improvements in attentional ability, as well as decreased depression. Effects on anxiety were mixed. Anxiety that resulted from exercise mimicked the anxiety that can result from psychostimulants. A low tolerance for exercise, poor cardiovascular fitness, or a high level of stress or anxiety could also be factors that affected this measure.[40]

Reduction of Medication

In another study, by Dr. W. Mark Shipman, many children were using medication. While running decreased hyperactivity and impulsivity in this study as well, the most notable finding was a confirmation of the theory that running made it possible to reduce psychostimulant dosages. Children who ran acted as if they were receiving extra medication. While the effects were most dramatic during the first two to four hours following the runs, a team prescribed medication based on daily performance. Doctors decreased stimulant dosages for a substantial number of student runners, even though the doctors didn't know who was taking the running treatment and who wasn't. As a rule, the more the students ran, the less psychotropic medication was required. After this study, children who stopped running regressed to old behaviors.[41]

On a practical level, St. John's Anglican Boarding School's physical education program has included relatively intense activities over the years. Students have played rugby three times a week and run three times weekly. In the winter, they have done 35-to-50-mile snowshoe relay races on weekends and, in the spring, have run 24-hour marathon relays. White water canoe trips as well as flatwater expeditions can take as long as three weeks in the summer.

Students have always been encouraged to go at their own pace, even in races. Canoe trips could take as little or as much time as needed, depending on the group pace. Winning was not important, although in this particular population many of the boys have been competitive. While such a program may not be appropriate for every child, large numbers of the St. John's students thrive academically compared to their previous school experiences.

While the program has evolved with time, St. John's still emphasizes the value of outdoor exercise. Students go on fall hikes for eight or nine days in the Rockies and winter camping trips for three or four days. The staff at St. John's still places a high value on exercise. When students in an assembly become unruly, they might end up going for a long run.

Non-Aerobic Activity

At this point, you've read about the effects of jogging or running on classroom behavior. We can speculate that aerobic activity, relaxation exercises, and meditation all involve deep breathing;

oxygen might possibly trigger the psychological benefits that follow. In any event, we can assume that any aerobic activity will produce the same behavioral effects as jogging or running.

What about exercise that might be too brief or not intense enough to be considered aerobic? A few counselors and teachers have reported that walking just a hundred feet can improve attentional capacities for some kids.[42] And the optimal stimulation study mentioned in a previous chapter suggested that simple calisthenics have a pronounced effect on cognitive tasks, problem solving, memory, and numerical and abstract reasoning.

In one study, brief, non-aerobic, large muscle exercise—one or two minutes of pushups and situps—has improved attention. The results are less dramatic than with running, but they do suggest that non-aerobic exercise involving large muscle groups will improve concentration.[43]

As a whole, studies that have looked at the effects of very brief periods of effort have been, for the most part, inconclusive. Researchers have tried using everything from hand grips to weight lifting to intense running to see how exercise affects cognitive performance.

In a few instances, simple math or reading performance has been shown to improve after non-aerobic activity, but overall improvement is not consistent enough to make any firm conclusions. For the most part, researchers looked for immediate effects and almost always used college students. Researchers have not tested these non-aerobic activities on children with ADHD, a group that might be more sensitive to brief, low-demand exercise.

Since weight-lifting results haven't been conclusive, you may feel that weights don't deserve serious consideration. However, some adolescents are more attracted to body building than aerobic activity. This built-in motivation might work as a starting point. Some adolescents who want to lift weights may not object to jogging if they learn that it helps with their muscle building.

School Programs

Since aerobic exercise can also improve grades[44], the success of the classroom studies might make you wonder why schools don't require aerobic exercise. (Some of the more enlightened physical education departments do require it, but, with only a few exceptions, classes are held only once or twice a week.) In a society in which schools are eliminating recess, exercise is obviously a low priority and is often considered impractical. As a rule, today's teacher is over-scheduled, overworked, and spends more time on classroom administration and policing. The need for policing, of course, increases with hyperactive children.

Working in a setting where many of the problems associated with ADHD surface makes teachers pragmatic. Although a few teachers have been able to use creative solutions to work exercise into a classroom schedule, supervised exercise is generally considered impractical in most school settings.

Nevertheless, many teachers and parents might welcome an after-school running program like one that exists in Kansas. Two times a week, children meet in a health club where they do warm ups while Tom Scott, their psychotherapist, talks to them. Afterward, they run in a park for 30 minutes. Some children run full speed as if they're competing, some slow down to walk, some jog, and some take short cuts. Running has effects ranging from a calmer personality to improved retention to improved grades.[45]

Flexibility is important for helping children integrate exercise into their lives—at home and in the classroom. If afternoon programs aren't available and schools can't fit adequate amounts of exercise into their schedules, parents need to supervise or encourage early morning exercise at home or encourage aerobic activity at recess and after school. How can parents do it?

Some Individual Success Stories

Encouraging children to play at an age-appropriate intensity is the same as encouraging them to work out. The only difference lies in the way you decide to motivate your child. Exercise involves anything from age-appropriate, supervised running to a friendly back-yard game of tag or neighborhood basketball.

Parents have used different schedules and different intensities, depending on their children's circumstances. However, scheduling needs to be a consideration. Teachers, parents, and children often have little spare time. And the actual time of day that a child exercises might determine the kind of exercise that will help with the desired behavioral and psychological outcomes. Here's how a few parents have helped their children incorporate exercise into their lives.

Mike was diagnosed with attention-deficit disorder when he was five. Now, in first grade, he fidgets and squirms in his chair. His teacher gives him the "thumbs up," a prearranged signal to let Mike know that he can take a walk. When he returns and sits down, the hyperactivity decreases.

Mike's mother, Beverly, acknowledges that this arrangement isn't perfect because eventually the hyperactivity returns, and medication is needed. When Mike gets home, Ritalin's rebound effects often make him irritable, until he goes outside and rides his bike for 20 minutes. Even so, Beverly appreciates the willingness of the school personnel to cooperate in meeting her son's needs. Large class sizes and liability issues might discourage this option in some schools, so she feels lucky that Mike has this alternative for at least a school year.

An elementary school counselor tells about Jason, a seven-year-old hyperactive under-achiever. The counselor had talked with Jason's parents and recommended a psychological evaluation. In all probability, Jason would have been diagnosed as having ADHD. Instead of getting Jason evaluated, his mother had him run to and from school, swim on a regular basis, and also participate in extracurricular sports. Jason's grades improved, and teachers reported that his behavior was acceptable.

John's eight-year-old son, Don, has always been energetic. Before he was old enough to walk, he had removed a heating vent where his father caught him trying to crawl into the duct. By the time he was in third grade, his teacher was constantly calling home to discuss discipline problems.

Don was getting good grades but was constantly fighting boredom. John considered a diagnosis to see if his son had attention-deficit disorder, but the principal suggested that the behavioral problems may go away by themselves as Don grew up, a common but often erroneous belief. John decided to wear his son out. They started jogging together and, in the winter, downhill skiing. Gradually, the behavior problems disappeared completely.

Early on, Don won a junior ski race and proved to be a natural athlete. Off season, he was running, jogging, and doing a paper route on bicycle. In season, he was participating in little-league baseball or playing soccer. By the time he was ten, he could run 6 miles or bike 20 miles. He was also doing light weight-lifting. In his teens, he could bike 40 miles in a day. Behavior problems never returned. Since training was so important, he focused on structuring his time and he also became more industrious. Recognition from peers, teachers, and other adults made him want to "live up to his image."

In high school, Don continued to improve as an athlete and was captain of a college Alpine team in Vermont where he also graduated. Today, he's a writer. He's no longer a competitive athlete and he doesn't train. But he still runs or bikes to relieve stress or, sometimes, to short-circuit his temper.

Some General Conclusions

Together, these studies and anecdotes show how exercise improves behavior and suggest possible strategies for parents. Ideally, ADHD children should exercise at strategic times. A 20-minute jog on Friday afternoon or an hour-long baseball game on

Sunday evening will have little or no effect on classroom performance on Monday. A 15-minute run before class would be more beneficial. Different ADHD subtypes and individual differences in brain chemistry suggest that optimal exercise times and intensities vary from person to person.

Regimens must also take into account factors such as age, life circumstances, and level of general fitness. For now, here are some reasonable conclusions that you and your child will be able to test later.

- Most of the studies mentioned here looked at the effects of jogging, running, and other aerobic activity. While length and intensity of a given exercise determine its psychological effects, there is a wide range of possible activities to choose from.

- Brief 10-minute jogs can produce immediate results. For practical purposes, a workout length of 10 to 45 minutes can minimize classroom disruptions.

- Ideally, children should exercise right before a class (*e.g.*, reading) where distractions will interfere the most with learning.

- In most cases, mild exercise will produce the most immediate benefit. Intense exercise might have fewer immediate and more long-term benefits.

- The most dramatic behavioral effects of exercise last from two to four hours but there is some evidence of more subtle long-term effects. Psychiatrists have prescribed less medication to runners, basing dosages on daily observations beyond the dramatic four-hour window of time following each run.

Observations on Motivation, Based on Studies

While motivation will be discussed in a later chapter, it is worth pausing here to summarize what worked in the studies. Needless to say, exercise won't work as therapy unless children can be convinced to participate.

- Adults provided structured supervision. In most situations, parental involvement is the best strategy for encouraging a child to keep running. Your child might not run if you just tell him to, but he will probably run if you go with him, especially if he is young.

- While rewards have ranged from ice cream cones to stop watches, most parents and teachers don't rely on monetary or material reward.

- Once they were trained, some children competed in road races.

- Often, children who walked or ran interacted with teachers and peers, in itself a small reward for some.

- Some children kept running on their own after the studies ended. Once a routine is established, internal rewards—mood elation or decreased depression in some instances—can become the reason for continuing. The fact that some children continue to run without adults or peers supports this view.

Additional Benefits of Exercise

Looking at behavioral effects makes it easy to forget the larger psychological dynamics of exercise. The chemical effect on the brain may be similar to that produced by Ritalin, but the overall psychological effect can be far superior. Here are some observations made by parents and teachers:

- Parents often perceive their children differently if they focus on the running (or other exercise), a positive part of life, rather than the hyperactivity that may have dominated family life before.

- Students who run also benefit from the encouragement of other students, parents, or teachers who run with them, and benefit from the improvements in self-image as distances increase and performance improves.

- There are more opportunities to participate in community activities, such as local road races.

- Experience is transferable. One student came in last and could barely finish a race; the police escort followed him to the finish line. However, the fact that he finished at all was a victory that the boy remembered throughout the school year. Later, whenever he had a difficult task, he reminded himself that he had finished that race—if he could run six miles, he could do other difficult things.

- Consistent with the need for a positive self image, a child can concentrate on becoming a better athlete rather than just improving deficient brain functioning. Young people value physical and athletic strengths.

- Even though exercise may not directly improve our self-management skills, making the decisions that lead to exercising probably do.

- Extra attention from a teacher or parent who runs with children might affect classroom dynamics. A parent who runs may become a better parent—for the same reasons that exercise helps children.

The Benefits of Excitement

As we have seen with rats, excitement or stress can trigger an increase of brain dopamine. While positive effects of aerobic exercise have been proven, the possible benefits of excitement also deserve attention, even if these benefits are somewhat speculative.

High-stimulation or extreme sports might also have some value, especially if stress and movement are combined in healthful proportions. Low-stimulation environments cause ADHD symptoms more than situations that provide larger doses of sensory input. Exertion and intense stress not only trigger the production of adrenaline and endorphins—nature's pain killers—they also trigger production of dopamine, the neurochemical that, in the right amounts, improves your child's ability to focus. A recent genetic study has linked a novelty-seeking personality with a gene that determines dopamine regulation in the brain.[46]

Adult participation in adventure racing suggests that this novelty-seeking personality is more than just a theoretical idea. Adventure races incorporate a variety of environments and activities, including running, swimming, ocean kayaking, white water canoeing or rafting, rapelling through a waterfall, and a host of other challenges. The race names, such as "Triple Bypass" and "Longest Day," hint that these races are not for everyone, especially children, but they do underscore the idea that adventure and excitement have their place.

This is consistent with Kurt Hahn's design of the Outward Bound program and St. John's Anglican Boarding School's belief that hardship creates character. As discussed earlier, in some ways, evolution and modern life have cheated us of intense stimulation. Thousands of years of evolution have prepared us to cope with extreme physical conditions faced by the predator, hunter, and warrior.

Now, at least in the U.S., technological progress shelters us from most of these same dangers. Most children associate food supply with the grocery store rather than the hunt. While modern life does present its real-life dangers, kids are mostly exposed to fictitious dangers on TV or computer games. In exchange for the comforts of modern life, most children seldom experience the thrills or neurochemical benefits of stress, danger, or excitement. Some miss this "adrenaline rush" or "amped" feeling, so they seek out inappropriate modes of excitement.

Excitement, combined with the right exercise, may provide one more healthful source of motivation for your child to begin, and stick with, exercising. One could argue that some "high-stim" activities are risky—and of course safety must be a high priority—but keep in mind the greater risks of immobility. For some kids, the joy of excitement outweighs the more simple joy of movement in itself.

Some kids need healthy amounts of sport-related stress, competition, or speed. In helping your child decide what to do, practical and safety concerns are primary issues that will be discussed in later chapters.

Consequences of Discontinuing Exercise

For some children, an exercise mix is more appealing than concentrating on a single activity. That was the case with Maria, who enjoyed a range of activities with her father.

For example, on St. Patrick's Day, Maria and her father would run in a local road race. In the summer, Maria and her father spent weekends hiking and swimming. Maria was not afraid to dive 15 feet from a bridge into 60-degree water.

However, after her parents' divorce, Maria's contact with her father became less frequent. On the rare occasions when they did see each other, they spent less time doing physical activities. By the time she was thirteen years old, Maria was experimenting with drugs and alcohol, and skipping school more frequently than attending. She has been arrested for shoplifting CDs, even though her mother could afford to buy them.

Any of a number of factors could have contributed to these behavioral problems, of course. Perhaps her actions were prompted by the stress of the divorce itself, or rebellion to get the attention she used to receive from her father. But it also seems possible that Maria's problems were partially triggered by exercise deprivation. One can only speculate, but it seems within the realm of possibility that the dangers of shoplifting may have been adopted as a substitute for the excitement of high dives into cold water.

Diverse Results

When planning an exercise program, remember that your child's needs are unique. Various sports or activities will work differently for different kids. Keep in mind that children who respond the most to psychostimulant drugs are often the children who are most sensitive to the effects of aerobic exercise.

For children who are on medications, exercise is always worth trying. It does no harm (if properly paced and physical dangers are avoided) and can have significant additional benefits in any child's psychological development.

Bob has a sub-type of ADHD that doesn't affect eye-hand coordination or interfere with success in group sports. But Bob has never had any luck with either psychostimulants *or* endurance sports in treating his hyperactivity. An auditory-processing disorder makes it hard for him to recall what he hears. He describes himself as "serious," and is depressed from time to time. Psychologists and psychiatrists have always encouraged him to exercise to calm down, but when he runs or participates in any endurance sport, he finds himself concentrating on the pain and boredom of repetitive move-ment. Although Bob would rather ride a mountain bike through the woods than ride a road bike on a highway, even a mountain bike quickly lost its fascination.

Although Bob never enjoyed endurance sports, he was an outstanding athlete while growing up. He does remember being afraid that he wouldn't understand hand signals while batting in a baseball game, and that it took three times longer than most for him to learn a soccer play. But he was the best once he learned it, because he was driven. At an awards ceremony, his soccer coach claimed that Bob could run through a brick wall if he had to.

Although Bob was highly motivated in competitive sports, he is not aware of any psychological change from running or biking. It is possible that he didn't run long or hard enough to experience any effects. But his situation was consistent with some other cases. Those who don't respond to psychostimulants are often less sensitive to endurance activities as well.

In any event, Bob's self-image boost from a great game lasted longer than the effects from a game that didn't go well. For Bob, exercise had different effects that were still positive.

Do these studies and anecdotes from parents provide enough reason to accept exercise as a viable treatment option for restless children with marathon minds? Many teachers and therapists who work with children every day report the same psychological improvements in attention span and self-image that researchers observe in more formal settings.

While improved behavior makes life easier for parents and teachers, there are often other benefits for the children. Think of the energy wasted by just trying to combat restlessness or live with a self-image based on reprimands.

Just as stimulant medication produces mixed results for different people,[47] so does exercise. The fact that exercise improves Bob's self esteem without reducing his hyperactivity underscores the differences from one person to the next.

Given the variation in effects and benefits, a child's exercise program should fit his or her needs both in the choice of exercise and the way it is evaluated. In most cases, exercise will reduce a child's hyperactivity. However, if it doesn't have that effect, but does enhance the child's self esteem, it's not a failed experiment.

At this point, start thinking about what kind of exercise you might do with your child. Think about activities that you and/or your child are already involved in. For the moment, look for obvious options. While thinking about it, you can always take your child for a hike in the woods or a walk in the park.

Exercise and Family Dynamics
5

The more I teach you, the less you learn. . . .

—Folk Saying

A chief was the only one in the tribe who carried a stone axe that was passed from generation to generation. The age-old custom lasted until the 20th century, when missionaries came along and gave mass-produced steel-headed axes to each tribal member.

Most likely, the missionaries intended to promote the concept that teamwork will make firewood-cutting more efficient. But the axe lost its value as a status symbol once every member of the tribe owned one. There were more power struggles, and the chief lost his status.

Small changes have powerful impacts on ways that families or tribes operate. What kind of changes will exercise trigger in your family?

Family Dynamics

While focusing on the value of exercise, it's easy to forget that the psychological dynamics of exercise also affect mental health. Motivating your child to exercise might be a complicated family dynamic in itself. Here are a few ways that dynamics worked in some of the situations already mentioned in previous chapters. Note that, in some ways, they resemble Jaak Panksepp's idea of "Rough and Tumble" play.

● Play can promote equality in a neutral domain. In the past, St. John's Anglican School has allowed "rowdies," sessions at which students were allowed to rough-house with each other and with faculty members.

Today, many parents would likely consider these kinds of activities to be questionable. However, at least at the time, school administrators believed that "rowdies" created a sense of equality for students and teachers who participated, as well as respect for students and teachers who opted not to. "Rowdies" took place only in a designated room, so teachers or students who avoided the room avoided the rowdy behavior as well.

● More recently, this dynamic was also expressed in hay rides, during which students and faculty who chose to ride in the back could push each other off the wagon into the snow. These kinds of rough-and-tumble, "king-of-the-hill"-type games don't qualify as legitimate exercise. However, at least in the context of this particular school, such games helped to encourage a spirited, mischievous, work-hard, play-hard attitude that made the children more receptive to the more disciplined activities.

● Consider the "rowdy" concept in situations where the rough-housing is psychological rather than physical. Obviously, joking or pushing for more performance needs the approval of both parent and child. Anything that resembles hazing is not acceptable, but parents can sometimes allow their children to have the upper hand—especially if clear boundaries are drawn. A child's acceptable joke on the tennis court might be unacceptable at home.

● Be the coach—if your child is willing to let you. John's exercise with his son Don, the competitive skier, was mostly structured. John planned most activities, a situation that might make some children rebellious or oppositional. In this case, however, Don usually wanted to exercise longer and harder than his father had planned. In time, he was also working with a private coach.

● Show your commitment to exercise. By running with her students, Jill Allen was showing them that she was committed to the program. It also allowed positive communication between students and teacher. While jogging, all were equals. Children like participating with an adult, and enjoy the opportunity to jog and talk with the teacher in a one-to-one, non-threatening situation. Informal support from teachers and from other students helped children relax. The school day began with a positive experience, and the children looked forward to it.

● Recognize your child's accomplishments. In his study, Mark Shipman reported instances in which "parents became more positively identified with their children's running. We saw success stories spring out of repeated histories of pessimism, non-accomplishment, and defeat . . . ."[41]

● Respect your child's individuality. Tom Scott, the therapist who takes children running, offers them individual encouragement while allowing them to run in different directions, at their own pace.

● Sometimes, it is useful to allow the child to take charge and play the role of the parent. An example would be the case of a father tried to teach his twelve-year-old daughter how to paddle stern—the back of the canoe—even though she weighed significantly less than he did.

After a week of nagging and arguing, the father decided to give up and keep quiet. The canoe zig-zagged like a rudderless cruise ship until the daughter figured out when to call the paddle switches and how to make the corrective strokes that kept the boat going straight.

In time, she became like a hyperactive parent, sitting in the stern, calling "huts" to make her father switch. He had to paddle to her standards or she would yell "Pay attention," "Pick it up," or "Come on." When they trained, she wouldn't stand for finishing a two-minute sprint five seconds early. As navigator and pace setter, she was functioning as if she were the parent. Today, she is an assistant crew coach at a major university.

New family activities can make some of these dynamics more noticeable. Your child can try new roles with parents or peers or try going solo, a more independent role. This depends on the child's age, sport, and other circumstances. Just keep an eye on how things are going from the beginning.

Positive and Negative Dynamics

Here are a few scenarios that involve different family dynamics at work. Let's keep it hypothetical for now, by choosing a sport that is not common in the U.S., pulling of rickshas. Here are some possible scenarios; perhaps one of them represents the general dynamics of your family:

- You sit in a ricksha while your son or daughter pulls it through the city streets. You get to perform your "parental responsibilities" as your child's coach and enjoy the scenery as well.

- Your child rides the ricksha and makes you pull.

- You and your child peddle a ricksha built for two.

- You and your child race against one another, each pulling your own ricksha.

Each family has its own dynamics—healthy, dysfunctional, or otherwise. If all kids were one age and had the same personalities, interests, and capabilities, then there might possibly be one simple formula for bringing them up. But even then, outcomes would vary because of the different ways family members interact with each other.

Family dynamics are life experiments that we can't always control. As a family member, you're so close to the interaction that you might not even notice the patterns, which typically involve conscious or unconscious decisions of who is really in charge, and how others struggle, either to gain control or to escape the power. If some of the dynamics in your family are not as positive as they should be, and you're the one who introduces exercise, you may have some opportunities to change things for the better.

As a parent, you may act as a nurturer, drill instructor, coach, friend, or uninvolved relative. Your attitudes, your child's attitudes, and your awareness of family dynamics might help determine how you approach this. If your child is feeling resentful about receiving constant, though well-meaning, supervision from you (and perhaps from teachers and bus drivers, among others), then she or he may not welcome a boot-camp-like exercise routine at six in the morning or four in the afternoon.

If your son or daughter doesn't want to exercise, it's not going to do any good to nag, threaten, assign guilt, or punish him or her. An impulsive child who is impulsively criticized by a parent will, most likely, become more impulsive.

Suppose that eleven-year-old Bob is usually lethargic. He's not the type who's likely to go out for a run or a bike ride on his own. Let's also suppose that he is a bit impulsive and slightly oppositional. You've talked him into trying to run eight laps on a quarter-mile track, while you sit in the bleachers and watch.

When he passes by on the third lap, you yell out, "Pick it up, Bob!" You merely intend to encourage him but he doesn't see it that way. Maybe he's not totally warmed up and his legs hurt. Maybe he just doesn't like being told what to do. No matter the cause, he slows down to a walk.

Suppose that this makes you irritated. On the fourth lap, you yell. He stops. The experiment is over. If this kind of dynamic exists in your family, maybe you need exercise to manage your impulsivity. Maybe you should be running *with* your child to manage the dynamics. Or maybe you should consider going to family therapy.

The chances are, running with your child in a spirit of camaraderie is likely to be a positive experience. At least that is true if the child is seven years old and values quality time with a parent. Enjoy this time running together while you can! When Bob reaches his teen years, he may go through a stage of not wanting to be seen with Mom or Dad. By then, perhaps the threat of being seen with a parent will be sufficient to motivate him to exercise on his own.

Dr. Stuart Copans often makes these points to parents: "Never get in a power struggle where someone has to lose." "Love and hate are powerful motivators. But what you do out of love is much different than what is done out of hate." If you believe that exercise deserves an honest try but your son or daughter doesn't, it's usually not a good idea to push the issue too hard. If it doesn't become a sore point, then you can keep up the discussion, with a possible change of mind by the child. Pay attention to your kids, and to yourself. Sometimes you may be better off going for a jog on your own. At least you'll be in a position to better handle the stress of parenting. And sometimes, the child who stays at home will want to go along next time.

The dynamics that motivate your child to exercise can also serve as a vehicle for the development of leadership skills and goal achievement. Your child will learn to take charge of his or her own life, and not feel like a victim. And parents sometimes learn that children are more willing to connect or bond after exercise. On one occasion when John took his son skiing, the ten-year-old fell asleep on the way home, his head resting against his father's side.

Keeping a Journal . . . or Not

Most parents don't keep a journal of their child's exercise activities. But a journal could be useful for evaluating the benefits of exercise and it could have a positive impact on dynamics between you and your child. You're not just sharing a notebook, you're sharing an attitude. Notebooks are inexpensive and not imposing and might motivate some children. Consider the journal issue as a chance for you and your child to negotiate some new rules that might change some patterns.

Here are a few possible ways that you and your child might decide to use journals. No matter which option you choose, it should help convince your child that you're on the same side.

A journal can help you make reality checks. Some parents claim that their child already gets plenty of exercise and that it doesn't seem to control his impulsivity. However, most parents over-estimate how much exercise their children get. Few, if any, stop to think about timing, duration, or intensity. In this case, a journal might help.

Since children and parents often view things differently, a journal that records each point of view might be interesting. For example, a father and his fourteen-year-old daughter drive to the river for canoe training. On the way, they have a ritualized, frustrating dialogue. The father asks how school was. The daughter replies, "All right." When he asks what she has learned, she says "Nothing." Conversation is impossible until after their canoe workout. After paddling, the daughter covers every possible topic from day-glow dental braces to disadvantaged junior high teachers whose sense of fairness never developed.

The daughter's reality isn't the same as the father's. He notices a profound mood change and describes her as less sullen and more outgoing. She doesn't notice any difference. It doesn't matter. They are both happy but view the same behavior differently.

Perhaps keeping a journal is just not your style so you pass, but your child likes the idea. A child can fool with recording heart-rate intensities, duration, or distance covered—whatever it is that happens to be of interest. She can write notes on why hikes aren't fun and why parents shouldn't impose them. She may enjoy monitoring noticeable effects of a workout.

In any event, the journal belongs to your child. She can exercise all she wants and keep the pages blank. She can write the great American novel or lyrics for a popular song. What if your child refuses to keep a training log, but uses the journal to try to complete Beethoven's Unfinished Symphony? That's all right too, unless you're one of those authoritarians who want to impose rock 'n roll.

For some children, an unscientific journal with ideas might be more valuable than accurate records. For others, ideas, insights, and moods can be a valuable contribution to setting up an exercise program that succeeds. If they want, children can record how they feel before and after exercise along with what they did. Depending on age and preferences, children can use words that mean the most to them.

Perhaps your son or daughter may not want to keep a journal, but may not resent it if you keep one. In that case, you might get a little respect for not forcing the journal on your child, yet have the ability to keep track of progress in a methodical way.

Or maybe neither you nor your child wants to complicate things with a journal. You both feel that life is busy as it is and that you'll know whether this exercise stuff is working or not. By rejecting the journal option, you and your child are agreeing on something. Keep the momentum going. With the $3.58 that you saved by not buying notebooks, buy two Power Bars.

In short, although there's a lot to be said for being methodical, that shouldn't happen at the expense of making it an enjoyable experience. Not only does exercise serve the marathon mind, it provides it with a way to enjoy functioning in the family.

At one time, the St. John's Anglican Boarding School's application process provided one last motivational caveat that applied to every boy who attended. Boys had to want to attend to be admitted, regardless of their parents' wishes. That mirrors real life, where most of us take advantage of good opportunities only if we're motivated to do so.

What Kind of Exercise? 6

. . . Children with ADHD are usually exuberant children with an abundance of desire and motivation, but their inability to concentrate combined with their impulsivity, distractibility, and hyperactivity can sabotage their performance on the playing field. Put in simple terms, these kids aren't coachable.

—*J. L. Alexander*[48]

If you tell a child who doesn't enjoy sports to exercise, he won't know where to begin, and will probably resist. He may already have experienced failure of the worst kind. Team captains can confirm a child's anxiety about poor coordination by choosing him last for a neighborhood baseball or basketball team. Besides, who in their right mind would want to wait in the outfield for a ball that never seems to arrive?

At this point, your child has two obvious choices. He can subject himself to the torture of waiting to be last to be chosen, or he can quit participating. If you don't help your child choose his activities sensibly, he may give up and go through life thinking that he doesn't have any athletic abilities.

You can tell your child that exercise is good for her, but that won't convince her that it's going to be fun. And unless it's fun or satisfying or makes her feel better, she won't keep it up. Do whatever you can to help her discover an activity that she might want to stick to.

Your child might already reject exercise because of a bad experience with sports. Think beyond the traditional glamour sports—baseball, basketball, and football—and see if you can interest your child in less obvious choices that might involve aerobic exercise.

Dreamers in the Field of Dreams

Children who are dreamers need a good sense of humor if they plan to play baseball. Although baseball is less dominant than it was a decade or two ago, our society takes the sport seriously. In America, elite baseball players are paid millions.

Ball players who are good, but can't make it to the ranks of the elite, usually stop playing in adulthood. As adults, they watch the sport on TV and read about it in the sports pages. In some adult circles, not knowing what happened in a game is as bad as missing a catch was during childhood.

On the baseball field, inattentive dreamers are always a problem. They're bored, standing in the outfield waiting for the ball to arrive, not feeling sure that it ever will. If they pay attention, time drags. If they daydream, they don't catch the ball or—even worse—it hits them in the face. They always seem to be sitting on the bench, rarely getting a turn at bat.

From a baseball coach's point of view, such players are losing themselves in another world. Not only do they forget the number of strikes, outs, or innings, they'll miss the ball when it comes their way. No wonder coaches and backyard team captains reject dreamers. No wonder dreamers reject baseball.

Playing baseball long enough to find out that one doesn't like it has other consequences. A child who is not capable of playing well risks an ongoing social price, rejection. A good player who misses a catch now and then will be forgiven, but it's a different experience for the child who doesn't pay attention—who kicks the dirt or watches the birds or yells at someone who isn't the umpire. Team captains will remember who pays attention and who doesn't.

Medicating to Exercise?

There are, of course, *some* ADHD children with good eye-to-hand coordination, who can thrive on baseball, and who find that it offers an almost ideal mix of exercise and mental stimulation. Unfortunately for most kids who have a strong need for aerobic exercise, there's not enough satisfaction and not enough movement in this game.

But one thing in baseball's favor—at least for some children—is how it falls into the continuum of mobility and immobility. For instance, it takes a lower dosage of psychostimulant drugs to play baseball successfully than it takes to read or do math problems.[49]

Medicating to exercise—and then exercising to eliminate the need for medication—almost creates a chicken-and-egg question. Which comes first? An eight-year-old who *wants* to play baseball to be with friends may find medication helpful. Is your son or daughter coordinated but having trouble listening to the coach? Again, medication may be helpful. Or, for some, a good warm up—such as running—might make them more coachable.

Galley Slaves and Rowing Teams

A hypothetical look at history can illustrate how dynamics between parent and child can influence a child's attitude about exercise. We know little about the minds of Roman galley slaves, since no one kept a record. There were no psychologists on these ships using mood profile tests to see if the slaves were happier after rowing. But it's safe to guess that they hated it, because they were forced, by hideous means, to do the labor.

Compare this to collegiate rowing, a sport in which people compete for the chance to participate. The Romans used heavy wooden oars, unlike the ultra-light carbon-fiber oars used on a college crew's racing shell. Now, high performance is the key. In the bad old days, they added a slave or two to help pull each heavy oar. Yet the basic nature of the exercise is similar.

Look at the commitment required for collegiate rowing. Crews subject themselves to hours and hours of rigorous training so they can compete in a few 20-minute races in the fall and even shorter races in the spring. Ironically, some of these crew members are psych majors who might study the neurochemistry of exercise. While a number of freshman quit rowing early in the season, the dropout rate is impressively low for the remaining three and a half years. If you ever attend a crew race, you will think that these students are having fun.

The dropout rate was even lower, of course, in the days of yore, but only because crew members were handcuffed to the oars and a soldier with a whip forced them to continue.

For galley slaves and college crews alike, rowing is usually aerobic and sometimes anaerobic. Use of large muscle groups—those in the back, legs, and arms—requires that the body supply lots of oxygen to these muscle groups. Generally, these aerobic sports provide dramatic forms of psychological relief.

Without stretching the analogy any further, it's safe to say that some children think of exercise the way galley slaves did. Even if they agree that it will make them healthier, they'll never do it voluntarily as long as they have that viewpoint. If they think of it the way a college crew member does, they'll keep it up—not because it's good for them but because they enjoy it.

Seek the Ideal, but Start with Something

We have looked at the possibility that baseball might be too boring for some, and the fact that coerced rowing will not work either. Almost any activity taken up voluntarily is better than no activity, and sports that aren't aerobic themselves may include aerobic exercise as part of training.

Teachers are likely to notice that football or baseball players are more industrious during the season and experience a slump after the season. While these sports help some children develop motor skills and teach them how to be team players, there is probably not enough movement to affect hyperactivity a day later—unless their coach makes them run during practice sessions.

The ideal in most cases is for the child to take up an aerobic sport that can keep her working at about 75 percent of her maximum heart rate. Finding a school close by that offers rowing as a sport is possible but unlikely. However, there are, fortunately, a great many possible sports and activities to choose from.

Perhaps it would be easiest to start with what you have. Does your child exercise already? Does he or she have a bike? Do you have one? You and your child could save lots of mental energy if you take the bikes out, as long as you agree that going together is a good idea. Will you appreciate the exercise? Will your son or daughter mind having a parent tagging along? Is this likely to be quality time together?

At this point, it may be worth trying anything that has any link with aerobic exercise. If your child is not convinced that there are any fun sports, try walking, a good fallback activity, at least in the beginning. No equipment is required. Unless you're in the middle of a blinding blizzard or ice storm, almost anyone can go. Walking can be as convenient as going around the block or climbing the stairs in a high-rise or as exciting as hiking the Appalachian trail. Either way, your child's breathing will probably deepen and become more regular, with an increased pulse rate.

How hard your child exercises is not an important issue at this point. Assuming that your child hasn't been doing anything that's aerobic, brisk 20-minute walks should strengthen his heart enough and build his aerobic capacity enough for more ambitious things that he might try in the future. Low-intensity workouts can also help in assessing your child's current level of fitness. If your child needs to stop and rest when walking up hill, for instance, his fitness level will require a gradual build-up before trying anything more strenuous.

Walking may help you and your child realize the physical, psychological, and spiritual resilience that's possible with exercise. While walking, remember that your heart is growing bigger, lung capacity is increasing, body fat is probably decreasing, and mental efficiency is improving. Your child might claim that she doesn't feel any different, but there may be some behavioral change that your child doesn't notice, so try to look for clues.

A Checklist

Repeating for emphasis, exercise works best if it's fun. Your child doesn't need to run like a robot on a treadmill and doesn't have to train for the Boston Marathon or the *Tour de France*. Most people discover their favorite sports by accident rather than intention, so do what you can to make those accidental discoveries more likely to occur. Sometimes casual interests evolve into healthful obsessions. Here is a checklist of things to consider.

☐ Is your child competitive? Does she prefer solo or group sports? Does she prefer exercise at home, outdoors, at school, or at a health club?

☐ What is available at school? Physical education programs that offer classes on a daily basis are rare. Only a few physical education instructors modify activities to accelerate heart rates for 15 or 20 minutes of class time. In classes that allow participation in conventional sports, intensity is generally inadequate. Do intramural and varsity sports favor the best athletes or do they allow all team members to participate?

☐ Is your child coachable? Does he pay attention in team sports? Or does it seem as if he's out in left field when he's playing shortstop? Does she respond to directions? Can she easily translate the directions into the required effort? As a rule, team sports require more coaching than individual sports.

☐ Is movement constant, like it is in soccer, or sporadic, like it is in baseball? Is movement intense enough and prolonged enough to be considered aerobic? If the sport itself is not aerobic, are there training exercises that make up for that?

☐ Does your child favor sports that use large muscle groups or smaller muscle combinations that require more concentration and coordination? Does she like running better than baseball? What sports seem to interest her the most? Is your child well coordinated or awkward? Generally, awkward children find more satisfaction with sports that require the use of large muscle groups, activities that are usually more aerobically demanding.

☐ Some children require more excitement than others. White water kayaking, snowboarding, and mountain biking are in this category. While parents might justifiably ask why their child should be exposed to any danger at all, they should also ask what happens if the child seeks danger on his own. Sport-specific safety issues always deserve parental attention. When these sports are supervised by knowledgeable instructors, risks are minimal.

☐ If your child has mental health conditions other than ADHD, consult a pediatrician or mental health professional. Make sure that exercise won't aggravate a manic condition or chronic, severe depression.

☐ How is your child's health? Are there any physical limitations?

☐ Has your child already developed some strengths that might help make a choice?

☐ Are there ways to integrate exercise into your child's existing schedule? Can your child walk or bike to school? In some cities where walking alone may pose dangers to young children, parents take turns accompanying groups for the walk to and from school.

☐ Are you willing to buy equipment for a new sport or activity? If so, learn as much as possible about equipment before you purchase it. High-tech equipment, such as marathon skating skis or marathon kayaks, for instance, takes a great deal of practice to master. Children will often be better off using equipment that might allow them to have fun in the beginning without making a major commitment based on an expensive purchase. You can always help them upgrade later.

☐ The idea of choice implies choosing one sport over another. In reality, many children like to participate in a variety of activities. There's less chance of mental burnout or injury from muscle overuse. Some find that trying a variety of activities helps them make informed choices. A family membership at a health club could make a large number of activities available. Even athletes who specialize in one sport cross train. While John's son Don wanted to ski, he also ran, biked, went skateboarding and in-line skating, and played in little league.

☐ Consider the possibility of using a journal to brainstorm ideas with your child to make it easier to start out.

☐ Do adults or older children in the family already have an exercise routine? Would someone in the family be willing to help a younger child get started?

A Sample List of Aerobic Activities

After going through the above checklist, you may want to give more thought to the variety of aerobic activities to choose from. The sample list below is not comprehensive by any stretch, so add to it anything that interests you and/or your child. And again, keep in mind that almost any activity can be modified to become aerobic. In this age of extreme golf and extreme frisbee, anything is possible. Also, even non-aerobic sports activities may include running, calisthenics, and other aerobic activities as part of the training.

Hiking/Backpacking
Cross Country Skiing
Jogging, Running
Swimming
In-line skating
Ice Skating
Aerobic dance

Biking
Marathon Canoe
Rowing
Jumping rope
Calisthenics
Badminton
Singles tennis
Squash
Racquetball
Snowshoe
Handball/Racquetball
Treadmill
Stair Climber
Ski trainer
Elliptical Trainer
Rower
Stationary bike
Tae Kwon Do

Motivation 7

*If every newborn baby has an appetite for forward
motion, the next step is to find out why it hates lying
still . . . ."* —Bruce Chatwin, The Songlines[50]

A classic new year's resolution begins with a promise to exercise. In a week or two, the initial excitement wears off, and ambition decreases the way it would for anyone who is dopamine-depleted. The dust collects on the exercise equipment, proving once again that beliefs about exercise mean nothing unless you follow through.

You've heard the saying, "You can lead a horse to water but you can't make him drink." Helping your child to get started might seem like a challenge, but think about what makes it possible for marathon runners to go 26 miles or Indian adolescents to run 40 miles through the desert. For most of us, these distances and conditions may seem like impossible achievements, even with extensive training. But athletes get tired and sluggish just like anyone else. Besides will-power, what other kinds of motivational tricks do they use to keep going?

In the real world, what does it take—from a parent's point of view—to help children become motivated to exercise? In general, someone who needs to run is likely to be physically under-stimulated. Even though he's lethargic and almost can't bear the thought of running, he can warm up by walking fast or jogging slowly for 15 or

20 minutes. At that point, he might become more talkative, as if on a psychostimulant. This stage lasts roughly a half an hour. If this person keeps jogging or running at an aerobic rate, he can become euphoric after three quarters of an hour to an hour. By then, emotional and creative energy might become more dominant characteristics.[51]

Of course, reactions depend on the person's age, physical condition, and the type of activity. The changes in mental state occur on a continuum rather than in discrete stages. We start with lethargy, with high resistance to exercise. We gradually move toward optimal stimulation, which enhances our ability to focus. Beyond that point, with an intense or long workout, we are likely to gradually begin to experience euphoria. While euphoria is great for stress relief and great for promoting exercise adherence, once that state has been reached, immediate attentional benefits will probably decrease.

In most cases, parents need to think about motivating their children only during the early stages of exercise. As the levels of dopamine and other neurochemicals increase, it takes less mental effort to continue to exercise. In a few cases, if the workout goes beyond a certain length and intensity, it might possibly become hard for your child to put the brakes on.

At this point your child may have a neurochemical drive similar to the Indian adolescents who ran forty miles through the desert. Luckily, in most cases, the competing reality of physical fatigue should make it easy to stop.

A good workout should enhance your child's neurochemical balance to the point at which endorphins kill some of the workout-related pain. The dopamine should elevate the child's focus, overcome lethargy, and make the child more receptive to reward. The neurotransmitter serotonin brings a sense of tranquillity. Warmup and motivational tricks affect your child's neurochemistry, which, in turn, strengthens motivation. It is this combination of psychological and neurochemical events that makes exercise rewarding and effective.

Getting Started

A child who doesn't want to exercise probably won't be receptive to the idea that she's a victim of lethargy or sensory deprivation. Your first task is to understand and accept that the lethargy is genuine. Someone who has just woken up, or someone who has been sitting in a classroom or watching TV all day, is likely to feel sluggish. Your understanding may help your child to trust your judgment more when you start helping her overcome this lethargy.

Remain aware of the dynamics between you and your child that are at work here. Your child's age, personality, and the communication patterns of your family will be key to determining the most effective means of motivation.

It's good to start out with a flexible plan. Remember that after the first 10 or 15 minutes of the warmup, your child's muscles will be more elastic. Her heart rate will increase while her breathing will grow heavier. The warmup loosens the mind as well as the muscles. Expectations need to be realistic. Half-hour runs may involve walking. Walks that were intended to last 45 minutes might end at 20. Whether or not you notice any behavioral or mood change, focus on helping your child establish exercise or intense play as part of the daily routine.

If your child hasn't been exercising, she may be more vulnerable to depression, restlessness, tension, or distractibility. Such a child will likely be more responsive initially to exercise, noticing the improvement quickly.

If your child experiences mood enhancement while exercising, that in itself should provide motivation. Even procrastinators can be hard to stop once they establish a routine. If your child has successfully avoided exercise for a long time, that same persistence can help in sticking to a healthier routine once it is started.

Avoid motivational strategies that are destructive. While exercise can enhance mental functioning, negative statements do just the opposite. Avoid drill-sergeant tactics. Make sure that your best intentions don't become abusive. Nagging can make a child more oppositional. Avoid lectures. Children would rather believe that they are becoming better athletes than believe that they are defective and need to improve their brain functioning.

Look for openers—take advantage of dynamics that may already exist. If a child thinks that he had a part in the decision to exercise, the feeling of self-control and subsequent athletic achievement can boost his self-image. Encourage your child. Let him have fun. If you try to trick your child, he will probably sense it. If possible, it would be better to help him adopt the attitude of self-trickery. A "show off" for instance, might hate to jog alone but might love showing you how fast he can run. Daring, if kept within bounds of safety and good humor, can also challenge a child or adolescent.

Depending on a child's age, parental participation and support are often crucial. Youngsters might prefer running with a parent. In some cases, children who have less time with their father may especially appreciate activities in which he is involved. Older children might want to run alone, or with friends, or with other members of a track, cross-country, or swim team.

Bribery—a reasonable reward of some kind—might work if it doesn't perpetuate itself. Ideally, however, your child should experience some direct reward from the exercise itself.

How Much Exercise?

In any event, more exercise is not always better. Encourage age-appropriate distances and performance.

No matter what kind of motivation happens to work, here is a rule that parents may want to follow. Encourage a pace that makes your child breathe more deeply but not so hard that she can't hold a conversation if she wants to. If she's breathing harder than that, she's probably over-doing it. To exaggerate for a moment, running a mile with a 20-pound back pack will impair any child's ability to do anything, even simple activities such as tying shoes.

Some Motivational Techniques

If your child is willing to participate in physically active play with friends, or exercise on his own, that's great. The following suggestions are offered only in hopes that they might help you think of a creative way or two to encourage your child to start out.

You can expect some initial resistance to exercise from most children. Instead of relying on your child's will power to force exercise, try to collaborate in finding a few motivational techniques that will be far more effective. The techniques that are effective will depend on your child, your family relationships, and family dynamics. The list below covers a wide range. Some are age-specific. Browse through to determine whether one or two of them may be helpful, or make up some of your own variations.

● In a sports world that now includes extreme golf, you don't have to take any specific activity too seriously. Is running the only available activity? Maybe you or your child would rather bike, row, play basketball, or try ultimate frisbee—a sport that takes more speed and agility than its more relaxed counterpart, regular frisbee. Almost anything goes. Let older kids act childish. Let the younger ones act more adult if they want.

● If your child is young, compliment her natural ability to run when she's playing on her own. Have fun. Encourage her to play tag, or kick the can, or runners and catchers. Have fun. Go for a walk and do short sprints.

● A good warmup is an excellent motivator. A slow 10-minute warmup makes a 30- or 40-minute session easier. For younger children, warming up can mean skipping for a few hundred feet. For older children warming up can mean walking for 5 or 10 minutes, then stopping and stretching before an ambitious workout.

● Help your child set realistic goals. Encourage him to start with easy workouts and then increase workloads gradually. For some, half-hour walks may be the ideal. Others might want to jog or run. If your child is out of shape, make sure that his initial workouts aren't too intense.

- Seek variety. Look for scenic courses, such as winding paths in a park or woods. Look for shaded areas in the summer. Vary workout times, courses, or intensities. Juggle activities. Run for ten minutes, bike for ten, then run again.

- Help your child add an appropriate challenge to a workout. How long can she last on the treadmill? What age-appropriate pace can she hold for ten minutes? Set difficult goals or hard-to-attain, age-appropriate milestones.

- Alternate sprints with slower paces. Let her try interval training— for instance, going as fast as she can for five minutes then going at a relaxed pace for one minute. Repeat this routine a number of times during a workout. Interval times can be one minute on and one off or three minutes on and one off. Intervals can accelerate strength gains, and can relieve boredom as well.

- Athletes often use "personal best" records as motivators. To recognize milestones as the days and weeks progress, your child can record workout length, distance covered, or how much time it took to go the distance. Your child might have fun with an inexpensive, old-fashioned pedometer or high-tech, beeper-size step counter that straps to her belt. One manufacturer, Sport-Brain™, allows users to upload data from their step counters on to their website where they can analyze and compare progress of other users of the same age.

- If (and only if) your child sees weight reduction as a motivator, help him to understand that exercise reduces fat without reducing weight immediately. Let him know that it's better to weigh himself once a week rather than daily. Body fat measurement is more accurate than weight monitoring, but to be accurate it should be performed by a knowledgeable trainer or coach.

- Some children should avoid competitive situations. Emphasize the value of participation, particularly to children age 12 and under. If your child enjoys competition, bike, running and canoe clubs often sponsor short, fun races for young children.

- If your teenager is competitive, encourage her to join a track or cross-country team. Or do a road race. For a small entry fee, she may get a tee shirt. Let her hang her racing number on the wall.

- Allow your child to accommodate his idiosyncracies. If your child is impulsive, he can go out for a run without planning it. If he doesn't feel like doing a workout, suggest that he delude himself by taking a break and just doing the warmup. As his muscles become more elastic and his mind loosens, he may have an enjoyable session—even if he didn't want to do it initially.

- Look for alternatives. If the weather prevents an outdoor workout, what can you do instead? Aerobics with a video or an exercise bike at home?

- Create an atmosphere that values athletics. Let your child hang pictures from sports magazines in her bedroom. Let her wear workout clothing around the house. Remind your son or daughter of sports role models whom they respect.

- Take advantage of your child's predispositions. Does a consistent routine work? Is your child a natural sprinter? Or can he grind over a long distance? Is he highly coordinated? Coachable?

- Commitments can be more binding if you talk about them. Encourage your child to discuss his workout plans.

- Take advantage of available dynamics that might motivate your child. For instance, let your child exercise with children the same age who enjoy the same sport.

- What if your child over-does a workout and gets hurt or becomes depressed? Injury or fatigue-related depression are just warning signs that can help you and your child manage workouts in the future.

- Encourage your child to find interesting distractions. She can talk with an exercise partner or use a portable CD player with headphones. Let her watch TV while she peddles an exercise bike.

- Let your child monitor his heart rate by taking his pulse, or by using an electronic wrist monitor. If your child likes math, wants to be an athlete, or just likes gadgets, a monitor can be useful. Tracking the resting heart rate can provide some incentive to continue exercising—especially for children who might not feel immediate or dramatic results. Over time, your child can watch her resting heart rate decrease as she continues her exercise program. Heart-rate monitoring will be discussed in the next chapter.

- Interface a treadmill, stationary bike or rower with your personal computer. Your child can exercise in a virtual 3-dimensional world. Depending on the activity, your child can race against an electronic pace bike or boat, or possibly even join in on-line competition with other children.

- If your child objects to taking medication, allow him to skip meds if he exercises in the morning. If he exercises in the afternoon, allow him to skip meds on following days. This strategy would, of course, require the approval of your child's pediatrician.

- Journals can arouse intellectual curiosity as well as motivate some children. One child might enjoy describing her feelings. Another might enjoy making the necessary calculations to monitor heart rate. Another who doesn't care about psychological change might enjoy recording personal milestones. If the bother of keeping a journal is an additional chore that makes it less likely that your child will exercise, don't push this idea.

- Negotiate. It's okay to use non-monetary bribes. Allow your child a privilege in exchange for a half hour of exercise.

- Identify fears that might be keeping you or your child from exploring options. For instance, parents and children who overcome the initial intimidation that they may feel about health clubs might find the atmosphere and variety useful.

Motivation is everything. At one extreme, junior ski competition motivated Don to work out year-around. His efforts exceeded his father's expectations. At the other extreme, when Mike gets a "thumbs up" signal from his teacher, he leaves class to take a short walk. Motivation is often subtle and not necessarily fancy, expensive, or complicated. Your child's age, abilities, and personality will all contribute to your motivational strategy.

Most important, try to tune in to the dynamic between you and your child. Not only can it determine the success of exercise, but it also a key to good parenting. Be patient and ready to seize the moment when your child shows interests or inclinations toward constructive activities.

Biofeedback— Checking the Heart Rate

8

Having described the peculiar features of the formerly so much dreaded athlete's heart as being, so to speak, abnormally normal, we can now turn to an evaluation of its plainly "normal" counterpart, the atrophic, relatively inefficient and metabolically highly vulnerable heart of under-exercised or physically inactive Western man . . . .

—*Krause and Raab, Hypokinetic Disease*[52]

How do you know if your child's activity is aerobic or not? How do you measure intensity? Anyone could guess that ping-pong is a low-intensity activity that has few or no long-term mental effects. On the other extreme, a 6K road race can be so intense that an untrained runner would see more negative effects than positive ones.

People don't go through life constantly checking their heart rates to see how much physical effort is being expended. But monitoring your child's heart rate lets you make sure that the intensity level is safe, lets you gauge your child's effort to see if it affects psychological outcome, and provides you with another way to motivate your child.

Is it worthwhile to invest in an electronic monitor? These devices cost less than $70, a reasonable price if they are used frequently but expensive if used only once. They allow accurate measurement with the least effort. Some children might be fascinated with the opportunity to experience first-hand the mind-body connection—the ways in which mental activity and exercise both influence the heart rate. If you and your child share any enthusiasm about an electronic monitor, it's well worth considering.

But if your child thinks that a monitor is more intrusive than fun, it's probably not worth it. Depending on the amount of accuracy desired, you and your child can also monitor heart rate using palpation (pulse-taking) or by watching your child's rate of breathing. No matter which option you choose, it's worth understanding how exercise heart rates impact health, safety, motivation, training and behavior.

Optimum Levels of Exercise

Exercising at an appropriate heart rate prevents fatigue, depression, or sickness that might result from over-training. Some out-of-shape children might actually be working at an aerobic heart rate when they're walking. For children who want to be athletic, workouts at target heart rates allow the fastest gains in endurance and strength. A child who isn't interested in the ways intensity affects mental or behavioral improvements might be intrigued by the process of determining heart rates that can speed the development of strength and endurance.

When physical stimulation is used to enhance mental functioning, an effort should be made to keep it at optimal levels. Certain workouts or intensities seem to have effects that last longer than others. You have seen instances where the heart rate dramatically increases while running, and the neurochemical changes that were triggered last for hours after the heart has returned to a lower rate.

Physical activity elevates the heart rate during the workout, yet it conditions the heart to function at a lower and more efficient rate and seems to condition the mind as well. You can decide how effective exercise is as a brain trainer and should be able to determine which workouts work and which ones don't—if you have an idea of what your child's exercise heart rate was.

Life-Long Benefits

It may be worth digressing briefly to emphasize that the connection between mental state and physical condition exists in all of us—not only ADHD children. Developing a pattern of physical activity may help children for their entire lives, in addition to helping them overcome their specific childhood problems.

The following story from *Hypokinetic Disease* illustrates this by contrasting the resting heart rates and intellectual achievements of one person who exercised with one who didn't.

An 87-year-old scientist cut his own firewood, gardened, shoveled his own snow on a steep slope, and walked an hour and a half whenever he needed groceries. On weekends, he either hiked or skied to high Alpine peaks for as long as 18 hours. On weekdays, he did daily calisthenics, read scientific literature, wrote articles, and lectured. His resting heart rate was between 48 and 60 beats per minute.

A 37-year-old woman decided to spend her life in bed after her father died. She managed to stay in bed for 30 years. (She walked around her house once when she was 39.) In her lifetime, she worked at some writing and musical composition but with very little to show for the years spent. When she was 69, she learned to walk slowly and spent a few hours a day out of bed. Her resting heart rate at that time was 140.

The heart's resting rate decreases after regular exercise because its actual efficiency increases. It doesn't need to beat as often because its ability to pump blood has improved greatly. In the cases of the Alpine scientist who was always active and the woman who spent over 30 years in bed, mental efficiency seems to mirror physical efficiency. At roughly 55 beats per minute, the Alpine scientist's large, trained heart would beat about 28 million times per year. At 140 beats a minute, the woman's weak, atrophied heart was beating more than 73 million times a year, over two and a half times the rate of the Alpine scientist.

Along with these differences in physical functioning were the remarkable differences in mental accomplishment.[52] Of course, we don't know enough to be sure that exercise was the only factor, or whether the woman would have accomplished more if she had been more physically active. In an individual case such as this, any such hypothesis is pure speculation. However, the anecdote is of interest because it agrees with studies that have already shown a strong correlation between physical activity and measurable mental change.

Biofeedback monitors have revealed changes in the brain's electrical activity that directly correspond to changes in heart rate. For instance, an electroencephalograph has shown an increase in alpha wave activity after runners train at 80 percent of their maximum heart rate.[53]

The Mind-Body Connection

Exercise intensity is not the only factor that affects the heart. Psychological states also have an impact. Coaches have superimposed heart-monitor readings over tennis-match videos to show players which heart rate facilitates the best performance. Coaches ask players to remember what they were thinking during parts of the game when heart rate and performance were optimal.[54]

Nervous tension, tight schedules, family or school conflicts, or pre-game anxiety can also increase a child's heart rate. Pleasant thoughts or a relaxed mental state can lower it. The mind can control exercise intensity. In turn, exercise intensity has some control over the mind.

Taking Measurements

The mind's sense of pace might have been a more natural sense in the past. You could call it a missing link in the mind/body connection. That is why it is worthwhile to make some conscious effort at measurement rather than just trusting instinct.

You can ask your child to focus on breathing and experiment with different levels of effort. Try efforts that are about the same as walking at first, especially if your child is overweight or hasn't been exercising. Try encouraging a pace that makes her breathe more deeply but not so hard that she couldn't carry on a conversation if she wanted to. If she's breathing harder than that, she's probably over-doing it.

Pulse Estimates

10-Second Count	Beats Per Minute:
7	42
8	48
9	54
10	60
11	66
12	72
13	78
14	84
15	90
16	96
17	102
18	108
19	114
20	120
21	126
22	132
23	138
24	144
25	150
26	156
27	162
28	168
29	174
30	180

The beats per minute are six times the 10-second count.

You can check your child's heart rate or show her how to do it herself by using the palpation method. Put your index and middle finger on her inner wrist near the thumb. Or put your index and middle finger on her temple, in front of the ear. Count the beats while timing a minute. Better yet, check her heart beat by taking her pulse for ten seconds and multiplying the count by six. Since your heart rate begins to drop immediately, accuracy diminishes the longer it takes you to find your pulse. Pulse should be taken right when you stop exercising to measure it.

If you're not inclined to multiply numbers by six in your head, memorize the ten-second count for your child's target heart rate so you don't have to stop and spend time with the calculations. Also, keep in mind that, at best, your calculations are estimates.

Using a Heart Monitor

Today, the more progressive physical education classes are using heart monitors to teach students how to pace themselves, to compare heart rates that accompany different activities, and also to train more effectively for sports. Some programs use the heart monitors with lectures to bring reality to abstract ideas about health, diet, and stress management, and to spark an interest in math or science—subjects that some children often reject.[55]

A heart monitor can have a powerful impact on children. It provides direct and immediate feedback during a workout by letting a child know if the heart rate is too low or too high—without the emotional baggage of a nagging parent or coach. All serious athletes vary the lengths and intensities of their workouts either with a heart monitor or by making estimates of their heart rates. However, as mentioned earlier, if the monitor seems like a disincentive to exercise, it shouldn't be insisted upon.

Heart monitors work like this: A transmitter worn on the chest counts the heart beats and constantly transmits this rate to a small digital monitor, usually worn like a wrist watch. Athletes who don't want to interrupt their workouts to read the display set an alarm that beeps whenever they are training above or below a preset target heart rate. Children can keep their heart rates consistent by using the audio alarm to warn them when they're going too fast or too slow, or simply by checking the digital readout. Parents can encourage younger children to exercise at an intensity that's within a chosen target range. If they need to, parents and children can think of ways to modify games to increase the heart rate. The heart monitor might also be ideal for older children or teens who prefer to exercise on their own.

More sophisticated monitors store workout intensities. Later, data can be downloaded onto your personal computer. While more expensive, the ability to download and graph intensities that were recorded throughout the workout might intrigue some children and parents. Since this monitor records heart rate at predetermined intervals, it could tell you how much unsupervised exercise your child is getting alone or with friends. This eliminates the hypothetical need for a coach to run along with your child, asking every five minutes for a heart-rate reading, then stopping to record it.

However, family dynamics is a key issue in determining whether to use a monitor. If you buy one and make your child wear it, you could easily create the impression that big brother is watching, since this monitor recalls how much time your child actually spends exercising in a target heart rate range. It's great technology, but not worth the expense unless the child reacts positively to it.

Reducing the Resting Heart Rate

Resting heart rate (RHR) has already been mentioned. It not only reflects the fact that your child is resting, it also indicates his general physical condition. Over the time that your child continues to exercise, he should see his resting heart rate decrease. For children who might not feel immediate or dramatic results from exercise, tracking the heart rate can provide some tangible incentive to continue.

From day to day, however, you might see occasional increases that have no more meaning than the normal day-to-day fluctuations of the stock market. An elevated resting heart rate might reflect anything from excitement to dehydration to an over-filled bladder. It could also indicate fatigue, stress, or the possibility that your child is coming down with a cold. Or might even be the effect of caffeine from soda or coffee. An elevated resting heart rate may possibly be a sign that your child needs to take it easy for a day or two.

Ideally, your child should record her heart rate before getting out of bed in the morning, but she can take a "resting" rate in any other position and time—as long as she always uses the same method and approximate time when comparing her heart rate later. If you're likely to forget or don't want the extra work when your child wakes up, do it later. You can let your child sit for three minutes and record her sitting rate which will probably be 10 or 20 beats more per minute than her actual resting heart rate.

Understanding Heart Rates

The following activities are for children who show an interest in heart-rate measurement. For those who would rather exercise without spending time analyzing it, just follow the common rule of thumb: Exercise should elevate your child's rate of breathing, but he should be able to carry on a conversation during the workout.

1. Test how stress and relaxation can affect the heart rate. Your child can experience the mind-body connection by trying to control his heart rate.

• While sitting, can your child lower his heart rate if he just thinks about lowering it?

• Help your child recall a negative thought. If he can't think of something that makes him angry, he can try to remember an embarrassing moment. Help him check his heart rate.

• Ask your child to think about a more relaxing moment and breathe deeply. He could imagine himself lying on a beach or some other place that he thinks is relaxing. Tell your child to keep breathing deeply. Check his heart rate.

• Of course if your child hates lying quietly and thinking about controlling his heart rate, there might not be any changes. Irritation might even cause the heart rate to increase.

2. Compute Target Heart Rates. Checking your child's heart rate lets you know if she's pushing herself too hard or not hard enough. Your child can exercise at target intensities to enhance the physical and psychological effectiveness of workouts. When you see the computation examples that follow, don't panic. You will probably need to do only two or three simple computations to determine a target heart rate.

An energetic child who spends too much time training at 85 percent of her maximum heart rate will not be able to achieve a peak level of performance, and the resulting fatigue could cause depression. If your child runs at 70 percent of her maximum heart rate for

45 minutes, her endurance should improve, and her resting heart rate should decrease more than if she had maintained a heart rate that was only 50 percent of her maximum.

For mental benefit, you should assume that an aerobic intensity of roughly 75 percent is optimal—at least until your child tries it. She probably will experience more long-term psychological benefit from an aerobic rate and some immediate but brief benefit at a lower target rate. You can help your child calculate her target heart rate using the appropriate formula below.

• Maximum Heart Rate:[55]
Age 5-8 years, 220
Age 9-12 years, 210
Age 13-20 years, 200

• Target Heart Range
Maximum Heart Rate × 60% = Bottom limit, Aerobic Heart Rate
Maximum Heart Rate × 80% = Top limit, Aerobic Heart Rate

• Example: Sally is 17 years old.
  200 = (Maximum Heart Rate)
  200 × .60 = 120 (Low Aerobic Target Rate)
  200 × .80 = 160 (Upper Aerobic Target Rate)

• The anaerobic threshold is somewhere above 80 percent of the maximum heart rate, the level at which your child would be approaching a condition of oxygen debt, in which the child's muscles would start using oxygen faster than he can breathe it in. For all practical purposes, your child won't need to (and shouldn't) work out at this intensity level, unless he is extremely fit.

3. Make heart-rate comparisons. Your child can compare heart rates of two or three sports or activities. Walking, running, climbing a hill, or biking all qualify. He can also change the rules of a non-aerobic activity that he likes so he can remain in his aerobic heart range for at least 20 or 30 minutes.

4. Make accuracy comparisons of the heart monitor versus palpation and estimates. If your child has a heart monitor or if you can borrow one, calculate her heart rate by taking her pulse. Compare her calculated pulse with her actual heart rate shown on the monitor. Now let your child compare estimated heart rates with actual heart rates while exercising. For instance, she can do jumping jacks and estimate her heart rate. How accurately and consistently can she guess?

5. Let your child check on his usual heart rate intensity in a normal afternoon after school. Are there ways for your child to mix aerobic exercise into a daily routine? Are there chores available? How often does your child have a chance to climb stairs?

6. Notice the extent of heart-rate lag. Since the heart rate adapts to the body's energy output, the heart's rate can lag behind the body's current level of physical effort. If your child starts running, the rate slowly climbs as the heart adapts to this new demand. If he stops running, his heart rate will slowly decline to a level that's normal for the reduced effort.

7. Ask your child to walk or jog at a pace that's appropriate for his age and ability for an agreed-upon distance. A day or two later, ask him to do a 10- or 15-minute warmup, then walk or jog the same distance at the same aerobic intensity again. Does your child find it easier to go this distance after warming up? In a half-hour workout, is the last half easier once he's warmed up? Does a slow, easy warmup help your child exercise for a longer period of time or go a longer distance?

8. Try to track the changes. How effective is exercise as a heart trainer? How effective is exercise as a brain trainer? If exercise reduces restlessness or increases your child's ability to concentrate, and if it also reduces his heart rate, you and your child might be able to track some of these relationships between resting heart rate (RHR) and behavior in your journals.

To do this, your child will need to consistently do some aerobic exercise at least three or four times a week. Record his RHR once a week. A decrease in resting heart rate should indicate that he's working in the target zone.

If you believe that there were no improvements and your child didn't exercise enough to lower his resting heart rate, you could encourage him to exercise more frequently or to increase his intensity so he's exercising at an aerobic rate. In any event, You will be able to make better judgments about whether or not exercise is helping to enhance his general psychological state.

The Fun,
The Dosage

9

*Downhill running elicits physiological and psycho-
logical responses that are between those elicited by
level running and cycling. . . .*
   —Abstract, Journal of Sport and Exercise Psychology[56]

E ven after more study is done, predicting what the effects of
exercise will be on a specific individual will remain an
inexact science.

As noted throughout this book, the anecdotal evidence and the
relatively limited studies that have been done are extremely positive
and provide strong clues to predict the effects of different levels of
exercise. Taking individual differences into account, parents and
children can perform some of their own evaluations to determine the
extent to which exercise will help and how much exercise is optimal.

As parents, you may already have realistic concerns about finding
the time to make sure your child exercises, then monitoring results in
some way. If this is the case, encourage your child to play or exercise
for at least a half hour a day at an age-appropriate, aerobic level of
effort.

If you wonder if your child should be taking medication, or if
your child *is* taking medication, consult your child's doctor. The
doctor should monitor your child's behavior, using the same criteria
for exercise as for prescribing medication. For doctors who have
questions about exercise, a brief rationale is included in the appendix.

What follows in this chapter suggests (but doesn't precisely
predict) possible outcomes for different intensities and durations.

This is not to promote the idea that there is a magical prescription, but rather to promote awareness of exercise's potential at different intensities. As the chapter title suggests, the fun is as important as the dosage. No exercise regimen will help over the long term if it seems like an unpleasant chore.

The classroom experiments that showed how exercise reduces hyperactivity and improves attention presented an open-and-shut case; exercise is helpful. In these situations, where exercise meant anything from walking to jogging, the average number of behavioral and attentional misdemeanors in the classroom decreased by one half—for three or four hours. But of course, that does not mean the results were uniform for each child.

Detailed examination might show more of a bell curve, on which behavior of a few children improved dramatically, others improved noticeably, and a few showed little or no improvement. In other words, it's well established that exercise will *probably* help your child, but objective observations indicate that the effects are different for different children. (The same is true of drugs, of course, which is one reason why they need to be prescribed by physicians.)

How do you determine what is optimal? What kind of exercise, and how much? If things don't go well with your first attempts, what can you and your child change? If your child exercises already, you might have some idea of how it will affect his behavior. Studies have shown that exercise intensity can determine psychophysiological stress responses.[57] However, since no one has performed a large-scale controlled study of the precise effects of intensity on hyperactivity and attention, you and your child need to know how to determine what intensities and durations work best.

Contradictions in Anecdotal Evidence

For perspective, let's look at behavioral evaluations in mainstream academic classes that immediately follow physical education. Some teachers will claim that there are dramatic behavioral improvements, some say there's no significant change, and some claim that the students actually get more wound up and harder to control. Why the differences in teacher perceptions and individual differences among students? Shouldn't all teachers see the same results?

Meaningful evaluation requires that you know who the children are, what activities they were doing, and when their behaviors were monitored. Mainstream student populations include those who are well-behaved, achievers, active students, and so-called special students. All have different needs.

What's more, in physical education class, students could have played sports requiring little exertion, like softball or touch football, or they could have played a sport with brief periods of exertion, or they might have been participating in an aerobic activity. Even if you know what the activity was, you still won't know how active each student was during the class.

Are the teachers who see overall improvement basing their judgment over the entire class period? If some teachers claim that students are wound up, are they looking at the first five minutes of class? Some teachers say that it's not the exercise that winds kids up. It could be that children get wound up after other changes in routine, such as assemblies and fire drills. The same things might happen, in some cases, in the transition from phys-ed to an academic class.

As a parent, you are in a position to look at your child's reactions to exercise as objectively as possible. After all, you are the one who can monitor how much your child exercises. In doing so, however, consider the evaluations by teachers, as they are observing your child's behavior when you are not present—in a setting where inattention and hyperactivity usually surface.

Just as pediatricians make use of reports from parents and teachers in determining psychostimulant prescriptions, parents should seek out teacher reports as a reality check.

Universal Benefits, with Individualized Schedules

As we have noted, some children, especially those who are inattentive or hyperactive, may be more sensitive than others to the negative effects of bland sensory environments, and more sensitive to the positive effects of light exercise. But virtually any child who is under-stimulated and isn't getting enough exercise could become somewhat inattentive, hyperactive, or depressed. The timing, frequency, duration, and intensity of exercise all influence mood and behavior over time.[58, 59]

For children who seem to be functioning well already, exercise might provide a buffer against future psychological stress. Everyone has a different threshold at which inactivity starts to impact behavior.

Low-intensity, short-duration exercise tends to have a favorable impact on attentional and learning abilities. The short-term effect is excellent but not long-lasting. Higher intensities for longer durations reduce depression and enhance mood—depending on your child's emotional state to begin with. It appears that in some cases, greatly increasing the intensity and/or the duration of the exercise may actually *reduce* some of the benefits for attention and learning ability immediately, but *enhance* them over the long run.

Definitions of exercise intensity and duration might seem too formulaic or clinical, but keeping them in the back of your mind can help you and your child after you get started.

The information's greatest value lies in the number of ways that your child can mix different exercise intensities into his daily life. Would the neurochemical effects of frequent, low-intensity exercise be more beneficial than an intense session once a day? Would the ability to just move around—the ability to spend some time pacing in the back of a classroom, for example—be sufficient to help a child to calm down and avoid disrupting the class? If your child can't move around during classes, would a light half-hour morning jog make him more alert for the first few hours of the day—or even longer?

Some general principles follow.

Low-Intensity, Short-Duration Exercise

Low-intensity exercise at roughly 60 percent of a child's maximum heart rate is ideal for children who have been inactive.

Walking, for instance, provides immediate results and there is no chance of fatigue. It's a good activity for any age, unless your child objects. As an example of this, a therapist in Oregon usually walks a hundred feet with an ADHD child to help the child focus before beginning a discussion.

Low-Intensity, Long-Duration Exercise

This combination still involves the same target range of 60 percent of your child's maximum heart rate. A longer duration helps your child build endurance and possibly have more positive behavioral effects. A priest counsels a teenager while they walk back and forth in the church parking lot for an hour. Who knows if the priest intuitively knew the psychological values of exercise, if he thought that it would keep the teenager awake, or if he himself suffered from the effects of inactivity?

Aerobic Exercise

Endurance sports require aerobic effort, the point where breathing can constantly replace the oxygen consumed by the muscles. If the muscles are consuming oxygen faster than the lungs can replace it, your child is going to slow down. There are two ways for your child to regulate breathing at an aerobic rate. If you don't care to monitor your child's heart rate, she can push to the point where she is breathing hard but not so hard that she can't carry on a conversation. If you choose to use a heart monitor, an aerobic rate is between 70 and 80 percent of the maximum heart rate. Your child may want to experiment with rates between 60 and 80 percent.

You and your child might not want to bother experimenting with a variety of intensities and durations. In this case, your best bet would be to encourage age-appropriate aerobic exercise. As already noted, aerobic exercise seems to be the most effective intensity for triggering mental changes. Activities that involve the use of larger muscle groups might also be the best option for children who are less coachable or less coordinated.

Young children, age two to five, can handle only a couple of minutes of aerobic activity at a time but recover quickly. If you take them jogging, you will need to take frequent breaks. A child who is between six and eight years old can run relays, play tag, ride a bike, or take short jogs.

Encouraging the idea of play can help your child to work at the appropriate intensity without experiencing negative perceptions of exercise. Children who are between nine and twelve can play organized sports, especially if they emphasize participation rather than score.

Neighborhood games are often superior to organized leagues where the scores have much more importance. At this age, children can train to run three or four miles safely as long as the activity is enjoyable. At 13 years old, your child can train harder or compete in short races. This is, of course, your child's decision. Parents who push their children to compete often have outcomes that are the opposite of what they intended.

Also, keep in mind that many high school athletes drop out of sports by the time they attend college. Organized sports can, in the right circumstances, provide much of the exercise your child needs, but it's important to be sure that the exercise doesn't stop if and when the sporting events stop.

Aerobic activity is the intensity that is most likely to promote exercise adherence. The intensity can trigger the so-called runner's high and help your child to establish a positive addiction. If this happens, it takes more energy for your child to quit working out than it takes to keep going. In addition to the other behavioral improvements already mentioned, a positive addiction often changes other patterns too. Sleep schedules and diet choices improve, for example.

Aerobic Intensity with Short Duration

Brief periods of aerobic activity have immediate effects. A woman diagnosed with ADHD describes family life in the 1950s with hyperactive siblings. When the family got home after a Sunday drive, her father wouldn't let the kids go inside until they ran five laps around the house.

Another example is provided by an 18-year-old recovering alcoholic who would get the urge to drink while watching TV. To counter the urge, he would wait for a commercial and go for a five- or ten-minute run as often as five or six times a day. Ideally, a run should last longer than ten minutes. But as long as he kept up this routine, it provided the stress relief that he needed.

Aerobic Intensity with Long Duration

With relatively long duration, aerobic activity should provide benefits in mental performance that will still be felt a day later.

Again, an aerobic heart rate is 60 to 80 percent of your child's maximum rate. Without a monitor, you can check that the rate of breathing is heavy but still allows conversation. For our purposes here, depending on your child's physical condition, long-duration activity involves 20 to 45 minutes of brisk walking, jogging, or running.

Here's an example of an every-day occurrence that some parents and children will recognize. Fourteen-year-old Mary won't talk to her parents when they arrive home from work. To avoid their questions about school and reminders to do homework, she takes off for a run. Although she is unaware of any changes when she returns, her parents notice that she's far more willing to talk about everyday events.

Although a little fatigue is healthy, it is important to avoid excessive fatigue. Aerobic exercise should enhance your child's mood and decrease restlessness, but immediate or long-term fatigue can actually interfere with concentration and decision making.

Marathon-intensity running for more than an hour should be attempted only by physically capable adolescents. Building up to that level of fitness takes careful training and lots of rest.

High Intensity with Short Duration

Anaerobic effort is a hard-to-sustain level and creates an almost immediate oxygen debt, so frequent stops to rest are necessary. Some research suggests that brief anaerobic bouts may improve learning ability for a short time. Overall, its practical value, if any, is limited— unless your child decides that it helps relieve the boredom of otherwise routine activities or workouts.

High Intensity with Long Duration

The anaerobic threshold in the 80 to 90 percent range is safe *if* your child is a conditioned athlete. This intensity might possibly be good for combating boredom, but your child should limit the time of exercising at this intensity. Over-doing it can actually weaken, rather than strengthen, your child. Immediate and long-term effects are mental and physical fatigue.

Heart rates over 90 percent of maximum are risky. Under this condition, the body has gone beyond the anaerobic threshold and is burning oxygen faster than the cardiovascular system can provide it. Elite athletes limit time that they allow themselves to train at this intensity. Children should never train at this level without qualified coaching.

Mixed Intensity with Moderate Duration

Defining exercise in terms of intensity might make it sound as if you should choose one intensity instead of another. Remember that games can allow your child to alternate high-intensity and lower-intensity efforts. If your child is starting out, she may need to gain the strength and endurance needed for a steady half hour to 45-minute pace. A mix of intensities also increases strength at a faster rate. If she wants to train at a more serious level, more sophisticated training formulas are available.

Psychological Intensity

If your child needs excitement, look for sports that combine aerobic and non-aerobic activities. Telemark skiing combines the excitement of downhill skiing with the aerobic quality of cross-country skiing. Mountain biking mixes thrill with aerobic exercise. White water canoeing mixes lazy paddling along quiet stretches and intense paddling in wildwater.

There are more obscure sports such as cross-country bike racing, a challenging event for bike racers because the required street tires don't perform well on grass or in the woods. These kinds of activities might provide an outlet for children who need more extreme stimulation than a daily jog or bike ride. Obviously these options require knowledgeable supervision for sport-specific safety.

Keeping it Enjoyable

Your obligations, at home and at work, and your child's schedule at school will often limit exercise times and choices. While a general knowledge of the effects of different intensity levels will be helpful, there's no need to adopt a clinical attitude.

Here are a few simple ways that parents have helped their children mix exercise into their everyday lives, even though they weren't always thinking about specific intensities. Six-year-old Mike fits in two five-minute walks during his school day and a 20-minute bike ride at home. Twelve-year-old Don bikes and skis after school. Thirteen-year-old Ben exercises on weekends.

What will happen next year if Mike has a second-grade teacher who won't let him interrupt his classroom schedule for a walk? What if he tries a 20-minute bike ride before school? What can his mother do to determine how intense it should be? Or what happens if he increases bike time to a half an hour or shortens it to ten minutes? In all likelihood, an easy ride in the morning may increase attention span and reduce the hyperactive squirming at his desk. And a harder, more intense afternoon ride may reduce the rebound effects of Ritalin.

Keeping Track

Exercise as therapy is more art than science. Thinking about activity choice and rules that might help motivate your child can make you forget the fact that excitement—which is another dopamine source in and of itself—may be the primary motivator to maintain an exercise schedule.

For some, spontaneity can be a critical part of a program. Eric was diagnosed with ADHD when he was seven years old. Since then, he has taken Ritalin during the school year as well as summer vacation. According to his mother, the medication worked well until he was fourteen. Though it seemed like a coincidence, he started bicycling with friends and, shortly afterward, decided that he didn't need Ritalin. To his mother's surprise, there were no detrimental effects on his behavioral or academic performance. Eric's experience proves that an exercise program doesn't need to be formal, complicated, or, for that matter, supervised in every situation.

Of course, exercise needs to pass the ultimate test; your assessment of how it affects your child. You have identified the behaviors or moods that could use improvement—such as hyperactivity, inattention, or depression. Now you want to know if the activities that you have adopted are helping. A certain amount of monitoring can provide the knowledge that will help to assure continued success.

Journals can be helpful. We've discussed journals elsewhere in this book, emphasizing that some children enjoy keeping them and others don't. Record-keeping should never be made a burden, but it can be very useful if it doesn't get in the way of the motivation to exercise.

If a parent and child both keep a journal, do their observations agree? A parent might notice dramatic behavioral improvement, while the child may not. A child may feel more tranquil after a run, even if the parents notice no change. Teachers have noted improvement while parents have not. No one is totally right or wrong. Different ways of seeing the same outcome might help you discover what works and what doesn't.

The important thing is not what *should* work according to the research, but what *actually* works for your child. Personal success can mean anything from feeling more energetic to feeling less restless. Since exercise frequency, timing, duration, and intensity all influence its effects, you can test a few different possibilities. Try using a journal or developing your own questionnaire to monitor your child's weekday and weekend routines. Which behavioral and attentional issues occur most frequently? When would exercise be most effective? When is time for exercise actually available? If children are taking medication *and* exercising, watch for interaction effects.

Record the length and intensity of exercise, and how things go afterward. Keep an hour by-hour account or just record impressions. Don't be disappointed if there isn't an immediate or dramatic change. If your child has trouble exercising consistently, look for more pleasurable activities that are aerobic enough to produce the effect that he is looking for. Stay with it. The addictive aspects of aerobic activity make it ideal for people who think that they lack the discipline to make themselves exercise. If exhaustion is a factor, find something that's less intense or just encourage your child to slow down.

Keep in mind the goals that you and your child have already agreed on, while helping him to decide if he should change his exercise pattern to get a different effect. Do you want your child to combine exercise and medication? Are you hoping that exercise will provide a substitute? How much physical activity does your child need for relief? Ideally, you and your child can keep the goals, and the measurements of progress, as simple as possible to avoid becoming distracted by administrative tasks.

Record observations rather than expectations of what you think should have happened. Report what you see, not the effects that this book suggests that you will see. If results don't seem optimal, encourage your child to experiment with different intensities and durations. Remember that you might find that your child is the same at home while a teacher claims that he is calmer at school. We all behave differently in different settings and at different times of the day. Also remember that what works today might change next year.

If your child dislikes the idea of keeping a detailed journal, encourage her to at least keep brief records on a calendar. She can record time spent, distance covered, or moods. If even that seems like an unpleasant chore, then do what you can to keep track, even if it involves only mental notes. To the extent that it can be accomplished without becoming a burden, record-keeping can help to determine what works and to revise strategies accordingly.

The following observations are not intended to provide diagnostic criteria for any psychological disorder, but they do suggest ways that you might note emotional or behavioral change. Some of these psychological states are peripheral to ADHD but are symptoms that can also be relieved by exercise.[60]

Hyperactivity

From the child's viewpoint, hyperactivity can actually be a valuable behavior, even in the classroom where sitting quietly results in feeling restless. The usual classroom problems—yelling, talking out of turn, leaving one's seat, disturbing others, or throwing things—may relieve the restlessness, even if these actions are also disruptive.

As the child grows older, he may quiet down in class. The teacher may be happier, but the child might still be struggling with feelings of restlessness. Parents, teachers, and the young person involved don't always agree when he is hyperactive or restless and when he isn't.

A journal can be useful here, or at least a simple record to track the effects of exercise. Also ask a teacher to comment on the child's behavior. See if she observes calmer or more attentive behavior on days when the child runs, for instance. This situation is ideal for blind measurements. Can adults tell which days he exercised and which days he didn't? Here's a list of behaviors that you might measure, to see where the child is in each continuum:

```
Hyperactive  . . .  Hypoactive (underactive)
Excitable  . . . . . . . . . . . . . . . . Lethargic
Impulsive . . . . . . . . . . . . . . . Reflective
Interferes/Interrupts  . . .  Cooperates/Waits
Restless/Nervous . . . . . . . . . . . . . . Calm
Unpredictable . . . . . . . . . . . . Predictable
Demanding . . . . . . . . . . . . . . Withdrawn
Explosive . . . . . . . . . . . . . . . . Tranquil
```

Attention/On Task

If your child exercises in the morning, is it easier for her to concentrate in school? If she exercises in the afternoon, does she complete her homework assignments? How do things go on the next day at school? If your child uses a psychostimulant, ask her pediatrician or psychiatrist if you can compare the effects of exercise and medication, to note the differences. The behaviors to observe might include the following, each expressed as a continuum:

```
Unfocused  . . . . . . . . . . . Focused
Inattentive  . . . . . . . . . . Attentive
Frustrated . . . . . . . . . . . . Patient
```

Depression

Depression can be one of the most serious problems associated with ADHD. If depression is continuous or severe, you should consult a counselor or therapist. But if your child is willing, it's well worth trying exercise, using different intensities and durations, to see if it helps. Some of the words used in the general mood scale are often used to describe depression. Let your child use his own words to keep a record. Some of the conditions that can be described as a continuum are as follows:

Interested	Disinterested
Excited	Lethargic
Strong	Weak
Proud	Ashamed
Enthusiastic	Unenthusiastic
Alert	Unfocused
Inspired	Uninspired
Determined	Uncertain
Active	Inactive
Calm	Distressed
Happy	Upset
Innocent	Guilty
Brave	Scared
Friendly	Hostile
Unshakeable	Irritable
Confident	Nervous

Intelligence

Exercise is a necessary precondition for proper mental functioning. Sensory-deprivation experiments have shown us how exercise counteracts the effects of an almost stimulus-free environment. Under these conditions, exercise improves our ability to concentrate, enhances intellectual ability, and helps us organize our thoughts. Unfortunately, the amount of sensory deprivation in these experiments was so extreme that it's hard to tell how much exercise it takes to enhance intelligence or academic ability in daily life.

Beliefs about the actual effects of exercise on the cognitive process of learning and thinking need to be approached with caution. Improved grades, for instance, could be an indirect result of classroom behavior or improved attention rather than exercise's direct influence on mental ability.

Unharnessed intelligence is wasted, no matter if the underlying cause of your child's stress is genetic or environmental (family or school demands). Intelligence is a complicated trait, and requirements vary from moment to moment. One minute, your child is searching his memory to recall the correct answer for a test. The next, he needs to come up with a creative solution. Some tasks require him to reflect on the past. Others require spontaneity.

Encourage your child to experiment to see if exercise improves her cognitive functions in classroom situations. Do small amounts of movement before or during class help? Does a short walk before class help? Did exercise on the previous afternoon affect classroom performance today?

Creativity

Some researchers suggest that aerobic exercise triggers creative thinking, clarity of thinking, fluidity of mental association, and synthesis.[61] Running, for example, can help some people look at old problems in new ways and become more adept at solving them.

You are in a unique position to monitor your child's creative energy—and whether or not exercise can be a catalyst. Think of daily problems that your child has to solve. Can your child find more solutions after exercise than before?

Substance Abuse

Because exercise can also be addicting, it can provide a substitute for the abuse of nicotine, alcohol, or other drugs. While exercise might not be a cure-all, it has been an effective treatment in some drug-abuse programs. Moderate aerobic pace and duration should be ideal. Obviously, if you ever suspect that your child has a substance abuse problem, seek help from a counselor or therapist.

Optimism

Here is another link between the mind and body. Optimists catch the flu as often as pessimists do, but—for the optimists—flu symptoms aren't as severe.[62] While your child can't always get what he wants, he's less likely to achieve if he gives up too soon. When the going gets rough, when life gets stressful, optimists don't give up. If your child believes that nothing good will ever happen, keep a list of negative statements that she often makes and see if exercise increases her optimism. Here are a few examples:

"I won't pass the test."
"No matter how hard we try, we will lose."
"I'll never learn to play guitar."

Self-Concept

Human beings are made up of mostly water—somewhere around 90 percent. This fact, while accurate, doesn't necessarily reflect our actual value as human beings. Most of us have conscious (or sometimes unconscious) beliefs about our self-worth.

Low self-worth or inflated self-worth can enable your child to avoid taking on worthwhile challenges. Self-beliefs can be modified by exercise. Since negative self-beliefs can lead to academic or personal failures including addiction, it is extremely important to try to keep them under control. Monitor your child's use of negative statements or beliefs that reflect his self image—or those that may be inflated in nonconstructive ways.

Deflated	Overinflated
"I'm worthless."	"I'm the greatest."
"I'm not as good as him"	"I'm better than him."
"I don't deserve . . ."	"I'm entitled . . ."

Striking a Balance in Your Approach to Exercise

An emphasis on controlling your child's exercise intensity and monitoring behavior afterward might suggest that you need to use a clinical approach in making evaluations. That's not always necessary. A few years ago, when John and his son exercised together, light-weight heart monitors were unheard of. Judgments about intensity were guesses. In their situation, frequent and often-intense exercise did the trick—without any further thought about what worked and what didn't.

The first and most important task is to try exercise and find ways to help your child to develop enthusiasm for physical activity. Monitoring does no good if it becomes a disincentive to exercise. (If the child says "I'll stop exercising if you make me keep a journal," then drop the idea of the journal!) You might find that John's approach works for your child, too. Perhaps, once the exercising becomes part of a daily schedule, your child will naturally find the right levels.

But that doesn't always happen. Sometimes it seems like exercise isn't producing the desired results, and the problem may have to do with intensity. Here are some examples:

● Your high-school-age child goes out and runs at race pace for an hour then tries to do homework, but seems more unsettled. Some calming-down time may be needed after intense activity.

● You and your child take ten-minute walks in the evening, but your child still has behavioral problems in school on the following day. In this case, the intensity of the exercise is too low to have an effect that continues after a night's sleep.

● Your child warms the bench in little league games because he's not a star player. In this case, he's not getting much exercise from the team sport and will need other ways to exercise.

Your ability to help your child will improve if you are at least aware of the effects of different intensities and have an ability to analyze the situation if a particular regimen doesn't seem to be working.

Meanwhile, keep in mind that all children are different. Some are more sensitive than others to the effects of exercise. And in any event, you and your child might want to reevaluate the choices and schedules from time to time. What kind of exercise is the child doing? How intense is it? What are the immediate and long-term effects? Are the schedules working out, or do they need to be changed?

Finally, it's worth noting that no matter what options you and your child choose, your child may welcome—and benefit from—your attention.

Risk Management 10

Like most things worth doing, though, risk-taking can be pushed to horrible extremes. . .

—*Sebastion Junger*[1]

Having read this far, you probably recognize how beneficial exercise can be. You are, I hope, enthusiastic about how exercise can enrich the lives of young people and alleviate the disabling effects of ADHD. But every good thing—even exercise—has potential down sides. How much "rough and tumble" exercise, for example, is appropriate? Some caveats and cautions are in order.

Many of the cautions—such as making sure that your child has a physical—may seem obvious, but it's nevertheless extremely important to keep them in mind. Once you start seeing the positive effects, the granola effect—the belief that since exercise is natural, it has to be good—can make you and your child blind to potential dangers. Please don't allow that to happen.

Concerns in Different Situations

The safety issues come into play mainly if your child is sometimes impulsive. A few of them apply to all children. Most also apply especially to older children who become involved in weight-lifting, endurance sports, or competition. From an athletic point of view, following the rules will generally help your child get stronger faster, and, if competition is a goal, more competitive.

Parents who encourage their children to do a certain activity need to become aware of the safety precautions that are practiced by seasoned athletes who do the same activity. Some risks are specific to the activity or sport. Canoeists need to know water safety. Bicyclists need to know traffic safety. Seasonal risks, exercise intensity, and exercise addiction should be of special concern to parents who may be inclined to push their children and to parents of children who may be inclined to push themselves.

For perspective, in some respects the safest thing that your child can do is to sit around watching TV day after day. There are long odds against the TV exploding or the couch collapsing. But well-being is paradoxical. To feel better, your child needs to take risks and needs to endure the minor pains and inconvenience of exercise. Excuses can make a mind weaker and lazier, so don't let your child use safety as an excuse to avoid exercise.

On the other extreme, however, confidence can evolve into carelessness, and parental vigilance is warranted. Understanding the dangers can avert a parent's worst nightmares. A ten-year-old swerves on a bike and gets hit by a suburban utility vehicle. A well-meaning parent encourages a twelve-year-old to enter a 10K road race—after the child ran a cross-country course on the previous day. After paddling a marathon canoe for 15 miles, a fourteen-year-old is a victim of sunstroke. Or a fifteen-year-old tips a canoe, forcing a cold and dangerous rescue in 34-degree water. Such events are rare but can be so horrendous that avoiding them is worth a great deal of effort.

Consult with a Physician

Other dangers can be specific to your child's medical situation. Are there any unusual conditions? Are there any reasons why exercise, at intensities that might be considered normal for others, could hurt your child? Does anyone in your family have a history of heart problems? Does your child have any allergies or injuries that could be aggravated by running or other aerobic activities? Most children are fit for exercise, but—to be on the safe side—consult your child's pediatrician to see if a physical exam is advisable.

Although the positive effects of exercise are almost magical for many children, it is not always the only factor in promoting mental health. Some children might also need therapy and, possibly, medication. If they do take medication, there's a possibility that the effects of exercise and medication can interact to some degree. The exercise may potentiate the medication, in ways that make it important to reduce the doses, for example.

Any significant change in your child's medical therapy, even adoption of something as normal and natural as exercise, should be discussed with your child's doctor. Reducing or eliminating dependence on drugs is a realistic goal to aspire to, but everybody is different, and exercise may have to be balanced with other treatment options. A truly informed decision requires consultation with a physician.

The Transition from Sedentary to Active Life

If your child has led a sedentary life so far, avoiding exercise may not only seem convenient, it can also prevent exercise-related injuries. Don't push too hard if your child claims to need more time relaxing on the couch.

Most likely, you're sitting while reading this. Your heart rate is probably fifteen or twenty beats above its resting rate. It's not ready for physical stress, and neither are you. The earlier chapter on motivation has already discussed how resistance to exercise can be normal.

A child who has never exercised regularly will need to phase into it gradually. There is a close parallel here with the need of anybody to warm up prior to exercising in an intensive way. Start with modest exercise—such as casual walks—and work up to higher levels as it is comfortable to do so.

Even after exercise becomes a normal part of a child's life style, warmups are essential. Not only does the warmup help the child to feel more like continuing to exercise, it also loosens the muscles to facilitate movement and prevent injury. Warming up usually involves five to ten minutes of low-intensity effort that increases heart rate as well as blood-flow to the muscles. The effort should be easy and relaxed. Your child should walk before running or ride the bike at slower speeds before speeding up.

Stretching muscles related to the chosen exercise will increase your child's range of motion and may be important for some older children who compete. Your child should stretch only after warming up or after exercising. Each stretch should be held in a comfortable position. Over-stretching, or stretching before warming up, can cause the same injuries that you're trying to help your child prevent.

If your child does an entire workout at a relaxed intensity that's below 60 percent of his maximum heart rate, there's no need to cool down. But if he works out at a higher intensity, cooling down will speed muscle recovery and reduce soreness. It also brings his heart rate back down to its lower range gradually. As you would expect, cooling down is similar to warming up. Your child can slow down for five to ten minutes before ending the workout. If she's involved in competitive sports, she can cool down while also stretching.

Age-Appropriate Exercise

The idea that activities need to be age-appropriate has already been mentioned in previous chapters. Obviously, this issue affects your child's safety as well as motivation. Children under six should self-pace themselves. These children need frequent breaks but might want to do occasional short spurts of aerobic activity. If you are exercising with them and listening to what they say, they'll tell you when it's appropriate to speed up or slow down.

Children between six and eight are capable of longer aerobic intervals—if they're in shape. Either way, self-paced play, bicycle riding, or short jogs are appropriate. Children between nine and twelve are more capable of playing organized sports. But remember that some children are less coachable and less coordinated for team sports and may enjoy individual aerobic activities. Children who are between nine and twelve can train to run three or four miles safely. At thirteen, your child can train harder to compete in short races, but only if he decides to do so on his own. Encouragement is good, but ultimately, it's good only if the child wants to do it.

Children who have been inactive may be more prone to injuring themselves if they try too hard. The same strategies that help athletes increase their strength can also prevent injury.

If your child is starting out, she can endure her first few workouts by alternating higher-intensity and lower-intensity efforts. In time, she will gain the strength and endurance needed for a steady, age-appropriate pace. Encourage her to walk for five or ten minutes, then do a slow jog for as long as she can stand it. When she's out of breath or her muscles hurt, she should walk for a few minutes to give herself a chance to recover before jogging again. If she doesn't get bored going slowly, take it easy. A long, slow, half-hour jog is better than a few two-minute sprints. (Although running is often used as an example in this book, remember that all of the same principles apply to any sport or activity.)

Avoid a pace that's too easy, but also avoid intense effort that makes your child gasp for air. Rubbery muscles and light-headedness are signs that she's overdoing it. Lameness afterward, extreme fatigue, or depression on the following day are indications that your child is trying too hard too soon. At the end of the workout, she should slow her pace to cool down.

To avoid injury and fatigue, your child should also balance exercise demands with her abilities and workload at school. There may be times when it is best to work out at a very low intensity or skip a workout. Severe pain means that it's time to take a day off to rest and allow your child's joints or muscles to heal. Or suggest that she cross train using muscles that aren't injured. (As an example, your child can probably bike if she hurt herself running, or run if she hurt herself biking.)

121

Watching a heart monitor not only helps your child maintain an adequate rate, it also helps him exercise at a safe intensity. A rate that's too low suggests that he's not pushing himself hard enough to achieve any physical or mental benefits. If he pushes too hard he won't build strength or endurance and his mood may actually suffer.

There is no specific heart rate that has magic results for everyone. Assuming that your child is already fit, working out at rates between 60 and 80 percent seems to be the point where he can get the most psychological benefit without over-stressing himself. While competitive training programs involve conservative use of higher intensities, increased intensity can result in fatigue and negative mood. More sophisticated training formulas are available for children who want to train at a serious level.

Signs of over-training include a resting pulse that's 20 percent higher than normal, concentrated yellow urine, or a sudden weight loss of four percent or more. Mild depression and lethargy are not only signs of stress but can also be signs of poor diet or overtraining.

Safety is also related to season and climate. Both heat and dehydration can cause muscle cramps, heat exhaustion, or heat stroke. Heat cramps are often the result of salt deficiency, while dehydration can cause heat exhaustion, a condition indicated by dizziness, headache, stomach cramps, nausea, or vomiting. Heat exhaustion is accompanied by a drop in body temperature.

Heat stroke is more serious. The body loses its ability to cool itself, body temperature increases, and sweating stops. This more severe condition can be fatal. In addition to the symptoms of heat exhaustion, heat stroke can include diarrhea, disorientation, and unconsciousness.[63]

Children are more vulnerable to dehydration and heat than adults. However, exercise is safe if they follow these rules:

1. Children should be drinking fluids all day—not just before and during the workout.

2. On hot summer days, children should exercise early or late in the day when it's cooler. Find a shady place to exercise mid-day, or swim.

3. Children should use sun screen and wear a hat and loose fitting, light clothing.

4. Children should never over-dress to sweat and lose weight. Not only is it dangerous, it's an ineffective weight-loss method. A dehydrated child will regain weight after becoming fully hydrated again.

5. Children who exercise outdoors in the winter need to dress warmly to prevent hypothermia. This condition is the opposite of heatstroke but just as deadly. Extreme examples would be an icy swim after overturning a canoe or breaking through the ice when skating. But there are more commonplace situations too. Perhaps your child is sweating, then becomes cold when it starts raining. Or your cross-country skier wearing light clothing gets cold when the temperature drops and the wind picks up.

6. In cold weather, cotton is not always the ideal fabric. Hi-tech synthetic fabrics allow moisture to "wick out," and breathable nylon shells protect your child from the wind and rain. Dressing in layers also prepares your child to adapt to changes in the weather.

Sport-Specific Safety

Parents need to remember that some safety rules are sport-specific. Some activities will require further investigation. Books and magazines are a start. Some running, biking and canoeing clubs encourage participation by children and adolescents. Members are often more than happy to help you and your child get started.

In the meantime, here are a few examples of sport-specific safety issues. Runners and bicyclists might encounter traffic or, in the winter, icy pavement. Bikes lose traction on wet leaves and wet center lines on the road. Bike riding requires helmets and knowledge of traffic-safety rules. Exercising in groups or with a parent is safer than taking a lone run through the park. For canoeists and kayakers, water safety involves using life jackets, and, in some cases, wet suits. Children who take on a more extreme sport such as mountain biking or white water kayaking need to be accompanied by experienced adults. Some sports have certified instructors.

Euphoria: The Benefits and Dangers

While unlikely, parents should watch for signs of exercise addiction. Euphoria—the runner's high—makes exercise more fun and makes it less challenging to exercise at a consistently high level. But euphoria can be detrimental when it becomes the only reason to exercise. Addiction doesn't always involve drug or alcohol use. A person's involvement with an activity or substance determines whether or not it's a problem.[64,65]

A positive addiction supports your child psychologically and physiologically. A negative exercise addiction can make him physically and psychologically weaker.

The line between a positive and negative addiction is thin. Immediate effects of over-exercise may be relief, while long-term effects include fatigue, lethargy, and inability to concentrate. These are among the conditions that you were hoping that exercise would help alleviate.

Your child may insist on running when he's injured and needs a rest. If he can't skip exercise for 24 or 36 hours without feeling guilty, anxious, restless, and/or irritable, he may be addicted. How can you tell if your child's addiction has become negative? Exercise should relieve stress or other symptoms, not add to it.

But if your child is addiction-prone, exercise may not be his worst problem. You might encourage him to start competing. Competition might motivate him to measure performance and plan workouts to help control his exercise schedule. As with any addiction, there may be other contributing factors. While exercise is a healthier option than substance abuse, you may want to consult a therapist if you suspect that there's a problem.

Most parents who are trying to convince their kids to get up off the couch and stretch their muscles won't face this particular problem. But it's within the realm of possibility that your kids may possibly become addicted to that natural high that comes from exercise. Up to a point, that's wonderful. But in an extreme form, exercise addiction can be dangerous, and parents should be prepared to recognize it.

Life Skills

As the term risk-management implies, your child can't avoid all sports-related risks but you can help manage them with adequate preparation. As an example: People often become dehydrated before they feel thirsty, so knowledge about a concept as simple as dehydration may serve them throughout their lives. For children who are attracted to intensive sports, lessons in safety may help them appreciate the risks that they're going to take and help them learn to prepare. Those are life skills that will serve them well.

Some Conclusions 11

What can we do? We were born with the Great Unrest. Our father taught us that life is one long journey on which only the unfit are left behind.
—Caribou Eskimo to Dr. Knud Rassmussen[50]

According to *Webster's Ninth New Collegiate Dictionary,* exercise is simply the repeated use of a faculty or bodily organ—exertion for the sake of developing and maintaining physical fitness. Sometimes, exercise implies a need to keep busy that takes priority over accomplishment—like the phrase "exercise in futility." Sometimes, exercise implies a need for self-discipline or external discipline.

Once a week, a boy hangs out in a college crew boat house, waiting for his parents to finish their workout with their rowing club. Once a week, the boy rows a rowing machine—without any coaching. At his age, he has never had to ponder or define the word "exercise." And his parents haven't had to think about motivating their child to exercise. For an hour or two a week, the boy lives in a world where serious exercise and play are natural. He paces himself and usually rows for 15 minutes or so.

If you spend time at a health club, you'll see the same thing. When the adults exercise and children are left to their own devices, the children start exercising, too.

To emphasize the importance of exercise for psychological enhancement, we have looked at its effects on behavioral, emotional, and academic improvement. Aside from the beneficial effects of exercise that we might see as parents, your child might enjoy a vast improvement in quality of life in a variety of ways. While the mass media have mythologized the endorphin to explain the origin of the runner's high, the idea of an opiate produced from within accurately describes the mind-altering potential.

Sometimes, making the point that exercise has mental benefits separates the idea from the experience. Any child who rides a bike knows what the hypnotic movement and accompanying breeze feel like, even though he or she will rarely think to tell you about it. What's it like to run a half marathon? Or paddle stern in a canoe?

Children who avoid exercise might be basing their dislike on bad experiences with a few select sports. Quite possibly, they haven't happened to try out the right activity yet. By helping them find it, you may increase the chances that they'll discover a nirvana that can relieve the stresses of riding to school on a crowded bus or the struggles with reading comprehension. Along with academic and social responsibilities, your child deserves to learn healthful coping strategies that promote long-term physical and emotional health.

In some cases, we may be reaching into the medicine cabinet before trying something as logical as exercise. For children who live in an environment where exercise is not encouraged or expected, hyperactivity can be a natural result. Ideally, the marathon mind should be encouraged to function in ways that allow it to adapt rather than be repressed. While there will always be an appropriate role for drugs, they cannot adequately take the place of exercise as a healthful, natural way to nurture the marathon mind.

A recent study shows that people who relieve depression with exercise are more likely to continue the treatment than are people who rely on medication.[66] Whether or not this is true for children with ADHD remains to be proven, but it seems likely.

Mainstream America Discovers Exercise

Whether we label children with a diagnostic category such as ADHD or substitute a more romantic one such as marathon mind, we tend to separate them from the mainstream. However, everyone seems to be striving to adapt to our high-tech "comfortable" environment.

Consider Riverfront Recapture, Inc., a non-profit organization in Hartford, Connecticut. In addition to a running trail along the river, Riverfront Recapture offers rowing, dragon boat racing, Olympic sprint, nd marathon canoeing, and kayaking. In 1999, its rowing program attracted more than 3,470 participants.

Consider the Charles River in Boston, Massachusetts, flanked by a running trail and a number of boat houses for area college crew teams. Consider the running trail that follows a creek in Boulder, Colorado. The trail passes under city streets to allow runners and bikers to travel without interruption. Elsewhere in the United States, abandoned railroad tracks have been transformed into bicycle trails.

Aside from the readily apparent physical and mental benefits, these locations enhance the quality of life for anyone who visits them by providing a brief and partial respite from the modern world.

Family Rituals

In the beginning, exercise might seem like just another chore. It might even initially create some of the stress that families always hope to avoid. But the rewards can be great. Exercising with your children can establish family rituals that will be treasured for the rest of your lifetimes.

Picture a Thanksgiving 20 years from now, with a visit from your grown children. You go jogging with your son, congratulating yourself that you're still fit enough to keep up—until he sprints up a steep hill, leaving you hundreds of yards behind. Pride overcomes the obvious feeling that you are getting older. You are able to congratulate yourself on the great job you did as a parent. Rather than stifle your child's right to play, you nurtured it. You remember 20 years ago, when you went running around a quarter-mile track at your speed, and your nine-year-old son took shortcuts across the infield at his speed.

Or you paddle a marathon canoe with your daughter, maybe with a few other crazies who think that the cold river provides a setting for an important part of the Thanksgiving celebration. Or you run a road race or take a family hike. The possibilities are endless.

In this hectic world where bonding with your children seems to require lots of effort, exercise may take you beyond the meanings in Webster's and beyond the science of neurochemistry. Perhaps you'll find, over time, that exercise routines have helped as much to improve family dynamics and relationships as to treat the effects of ADHD.

Nothing in this world is 100 percent certain. For any particular child, there is no absolute guarantee that either medication or exercise will help. You won't know the effectiveness of any therapy until you try it.

But the chances are very good that an exercise routine will help a child with a marathon mind to adapt to the society in which we all must exist, while providing many other quality-of-life benefits as well. I hope that this book has given you the information you need and the motivation to give it a try.

Appendix

Note to Physician

Available research suggests that aerobic exercise can relieve depression and anxiety. Some data also suggest that aerobic exercise relieves ADHD symptoms. In some cases, exercise allows reduction or discontinuation of stimulant medication. Parents are aware that the need for medical diagnosis, monitoring, and treatment should be determined by the child's physician, working together with the child's teachers and parents.

References:

1. Greist, J. H., "Running as Treatment for Depression," *Comprehensive Psychiatry,* V. 20, pp. 41-54.

2. Panksepp, J., "Attention Deficit Hyperactivity Disorders, Psychostimulants, and Intolerance of Childhood Playfulness: A Tragedy in the Making?" *Current Directions In Psychological Science,* June 1998, V. 7, No. 3, pp. 91-98.

3. Shipman, W. M., "Emotional and Behavioral Effects of Long-Distance Running on Children," *Running as Therapy.* Edited by M.L. Sachs and G.W. Buffone. University of Nebraska Press, 1985, pp. 125-137.

4. Allen, J. I., "Jogging Can Modify Disruptive Behaviors," *Teaching Exceptional Children,* Winter 1980, pp. 66-70.

5. Bass, C. K., "Running Can Modify Classroom Behavior," *Journal of Learning Disabilities,* 1985, V. 18, No. 3. pp. 160-161.

6. Elsom, S. D., *Self-Management of Hyperactivity: Children's Use of Jogging,* 1980, UMI Dissertation Services.

Endnotes

1. Junger, S., "The Joy of Danger." *Utne Reader.* August, 1998 pp. 58-63.

2. Panksepp, J., "Attention Deficit Hyperactivity Disorders, Psychostimulants, and Intolerance of Childhood Playfulness: A Tragedy in the Making?" *Current Directions In Psychological Science,* June 1998, V.7, No.3, pp.91-98.

3. Kelleher, K.J., M.D., *et al,* "Increasing Identification of Psychosocial Problems: 1979-1996." *Pediatrics.* June, 2000. V105. No. 6 pp 1313-1321.

4. Gainetdinov, R.R., "Role of Serotonin in the Paradoxical Calming Effect of Psychostimulants on Hyperactivity." *Science.* 15 Jan. 1999 Vol. 283 pp. 397-401.

5. U.S. Dept. of Health & Human Services. *Physical Activity and Health,* A Report of the Surgeon General, 1996.

6. Child's Right to Play, *www.ipausa.org.*

7. Jensen, P.S., M.D., "Evolution and Revolution in Child Psychiatry: ADHD as a Disorder of Adaptation." *Journal of the American Academy of Child and Adolescent Psychiatry* V36. No. 12, Dec. 97, pp 1672-1679.

8. Putnam, S. and Copans, S.A. "Exercise: An Alternative Approach to the Treatment of ADHD." *Reaching Today's Youth.* Winter 1998. pp.66-68.

9. Breggin, P. R , *Talking Back to Ritalin.* Common Courage Press, 1998. Pp. 74-78

10. Newkirk, T., "Misreading Masculinity: Speculations on the Great Gender Gap in Writing." *Language Arts,* Vol. 77 No.4, March 2000.

11. Women's Sports Foundation Report: *Sport & Teen Pregnancy.* www.womens-sport foundation.org

12. Berry, C.A., Shaywitz,S.E. & B.A. "Girls with Attention Deficit Disorder: A Silent Minority? A Report on Behavioral and Cognitive Characteristics. *Pediatrics.* November 1985. V. 76. No. 5. Pp. 801-809.

13. Dienstbier, R.A., "The Effect of Exercise on Personality." *Running as Therapy.* Sachs, M.L., Buffone, G.W. Eds. 1984, University of Nebraska Press. pp. 253-270

14. Bennett, Knorr, Copans, "Which of These Children has ADHD? The Answer Might Surprise You." *Reaching Today's Youth.* Winter 1998. Pp. 6-10

15. Jokyl, E., "Running, Psychology, and Culture." *Annals New York Academy of Sciences.* 1977. V. 301, pp. 970-1001

16. Zubek, J.P. "Counteracting Effects of Physical Exercises Performed during Prolonged Perceptual Deprivation." *Science.* 1963. V. 142. pp. 504-506

17. Zentall, S., "Optimal Stimulation as Theoretical Basis of Hyperactivity." *American Journal of Orthopsychiatry.* 1975. V. 45 (4). pp 549-563.

18. Kraus, H.and Raab, W. *Hypokinetic Disease.* Charles C. Thomas, 1961. pp. 145-151

19. Fry, R.W. *et al.,* "Psychological and immunological correlates of acute overtraining." *British Journal of Sports Medicine.* V28 pp. 241-246

20. Heron, W., *et al,* "Visual Disturbances after Prolonged Perceptual Isolation." *Canadian Journal of Psychology.* 1956. V.10. No. 1 Pp 13-18.

21. Solomon, E. G. and Bumpus, A. K. "The Running Meditation Response: An Adjunct to Psychotherapy." *American Journal of Psychotherapy.* 1978 V. 32, No.4. pp. 583-592.

22. Ferguson, K.J., "Attitudes, Knowledge, and Beliefs as Predictors of Exercise Intent and Behavior in Schoolchildren." *Journal of School Health,* March 1989, V.59, No.3 pp. 112-115.

23. Ratey, J. Interview, America OnLine Psych Forum, Third Annual National Attention Deficit Disorder Adult A.D.D. Conference in St. Louis, 5/16/97).

24. Panksepp, J. *Affective Neuroscience.* Oxford University Press. 1998 Pp. 280-299.

25. Olds, J. & Milner, P. "Positive Reinforcement Produced by Electrical Stimulation of the Septal Area and Other Regions of the Rat Brain." *Journal of Comparative Physiological Psychology.* V. 47. pp 419-428.

26. Shaywitz, B. A., *et al.* "Selective Brain Dopamine Depletion in Developing Rats: An Experimental Model of Minimal Brain Dysfunction." *Science.* 1976. V. 191. pp 305-308.

27. Yokel, R.A., *et al.* "Increased Lever Pressing for Amphetamine after Pimozide in Rats: Implications for a Dopamine Theory of Reward." *Science.* 1975. V. 187. pp. 547-549.

28. Guffey, D.G., "Ritalin: What Educators and Parents Should Know." *Journal of Instructional Psychology.* V 19. No. 3.

29. Rapport, M.D., *et al.* "Attention Deficit Disorder and Methylphenidate: A Multilevel Analysis of Dose-Response Effects on Children's Impulsivity Across Settings." *Journal of the American Academy of Child Psychiatry.* 1988. V. 27. pp.60-69.

Endnotes

30. Hawkes, C., "Endorphins: the basis of pleasure?" *Journal of Neurology, Neurosurgery, and Psychiatry*. 1992, V. 55. pp 247-250.

31. Koltyn, K.F., "Perception of Pain Following Aerobic Exercise." *Medicine & Science in Sports and Exercise*. 1996. pp. 1418-1421

32. Pysh, J.J. and Weiss, G.M. "Exercise During Development Induces an Increase in Purkinje Cell Dendritic Tree Size." *Science*. 1979. V. 206, pp. 230-231.

33. Bliss, E.L. and Ailion, J. "Relationship of Stress and Activity to Brain Dopamine and Homovanillic Acid." *Life Sciences*. 1971. V. 10, Part I. pp. 1161-1169.

34. Post, R.M., *et al.* "Psychomotor Activity and Cerebrospinal Fluid Amine Metabolites in Affective Illness." *American Journal of Psychiatry*. 1973. V. 130:1. pp. 67-72.

35. Ratey,J.J. *A User's Guide to the Brain*. Pantheon. 2001

36. van Praag, H. *et al*, "Running enhances neurogenesis, learning, and long-term potentiation in mice. *Proceedings of the National Academy of Sciences* Vol. 96, issue 23, pp. 13427-13431)

37. Hartmann, T., *Attention Deficit Disorder: A Different Perception*. Underwood-Miller. 1993

38. Allen, J.I. "Jogging Can Modify Disruptive Behaviors." *Teaching Exceptional Children*. Winter 1980. pp. 66-70.

39. Bass, C. K. "Running Can Modify Classroom Behavior." *Journal of Learning Disabilities*. 1985. V. 18, No. 3. pp. 160-161.

40. Elsom, S.D. *Self-Management of Hyperactivity: Children's Use of Jogging*. 1980. UMI Dissertation Services.

41. Shipman, W. M., "Emotional and Behavioral Effects of Long-Distance Running on Children." *Running as Therapy*. Edited by M.L. Sachs and G.W. Buffone. University of Nebraska Press. 1985. pp. 125-137.

42. Gerchufsky, M. "Helping Families Cope with ADHD." *ADVANCE for Nurse Practitioners*. February 1996. pp. 39-42.

43. Klein, S.A. and Deffenbacher, J.L. "Relaxation and Exercise for Hyperactive Impulsive Children." *Perceptual and Motor Skills*. 1977, V. 45. pp. 1159-1162.

44. International Society of Sport Psychology Position Statement. *The Physician and Sportsmedicine*. Oct. 1992. V.20., pp. 179-184.

45. Higdon, H. "Getting Their Attention". *Runner's World,* July 1999. V34. I7. p84.

46. Benjamin, J., *et al.* "Population and Familial Association between the D4 Dopamine Receptor Gene and Measures of Novelty Seeking." *Nature Genetics.* 1996. V12. pp. 81-84.

47. Garber, S.W., *et al. Beyond Ritalin.,* Harper Perennial, 1997. Chapter II, "Medication Myths." pp. 12-23.

48. Alexander, J. L. "Hyperactive Children: Which Sports Have the Right Stuff?" *The Physician and Sportsmedicine.* 1990. V. 18, No. 4. pp. 105-108.

49. Pelham, W.E., "Methylphenidate and Baseball Playing in ADHD Children: Who's on First?" *Journal of Consulting and Clinical Psychology.* 1990. V.58, No. 1. pp.130-133.

50. Chatwin, Bruce, *The Songlines.* 1988, Penguin Books

51. Kostrubala, T., *Running as Therapy.* Edited by M.L. Sachs and G.W. Buffone. University of Nebraska Press. 1985. pp. 112-124.

52. Kraus, H. and Raab, W. *Hypokinetic Disease.* Charles C. Thomas, 1961. pp. 61-79.

53. Boutcher, S. H. and Landers, D. M-. "The Effects of Vigorous Exercise on Anxiety, Heart Rate, and Alpha Activity of Runners and Nonrunners." *Psychophysiology.* Nov. 1988. V. 25, No. 6. pp.696-702.

54. Edwards, S. *The Heart Rate Monitor Book.* Polar CIC. 1993.

55. Kirkpatrick, B. and Birnbaum, B. *Lessons From the Heart.* Human Kinetics. 1997 pp. 8-10

56. Abstract, *Journal of Sport and Exercise Psychology,* 1994, V16., p.451 (abstracts article by Lawson, T.R., *et al. Canadian Journal of Applied Physiology.* V19., pp91-100.

57. Rejeski, W.J.,*et al.* "The Effects of Varying Doses of Acute Aerobic Exercise on Psychophysiological Stress Responses in Highly Trained Cyclists." *Journal of Sport & Exercise Psychology,* 1991. V13. pp. 188-199

58. Berger, B. G. "Stress Reduction and Mood Enhancement in Four Exercise Modes: Swimming, Body Conditioning, Hatha Yoga, and Fencing" *Research Quarterly For Exercise and Sport.* 1988. Vol. 59, No. 2 pp. 148-159.

59. Plante, T.G. "Aerobic Exercise in Prevention and Treatment of Psychopathology." *Exercise Psychology: The influence of physical exercise on psychological process.* 1993 Seraganian, P. Ed. New York. Wiley.

60. Hinkle, J.S. "Aerobic Running Behavior and Psychotherapeutics: Implications for Sports Counseling and Psychology." *Journal of Sport Behavior.* 1992. Vol. 15, No.4 pp.263-277.

61. Hays, K.F. "Running Therapy: Special Characteristics and Therapeutic Issues of Concern." *Psychotherapy.* V31. #4. pp. 725-729.

62. Kavussanu, M. and McAuley, E. "Exercise and Optimism: Are Highly Active Individuals More Optimistic? *Journal of Sport and Exercise Psychology.* 1995. V17. pp. 246-248

63. Clark, T., *Runner's World.* June 1998. pp. 71-75

64. Sachs, M. L. "Running Addiction." *Psychology of Running.* M.H. and M.L. Sachs, Editors. Human Kinetics Publ. Champaign, IL. pp. 116-126.

65. Sachs, M.L. and Pargman, D. "Running Addiction." *Running as Therapy.* Edited by M.L. Sachs and G.W. Buffone. University of Nebraska Press. 1985. pp. 231-252.

66 Blumenthal, J.A., "Effects of Exercise Training on Older Patients with Major Depression." *Archives of Internal Medicine.* Oct. 1999, V.159., No. 19.

Bibliography

Fiction/Anthropology

Chatwin, B., *The Songlines,* New York, Penguin, 1988

The Brain

Ratey, J. J. *A User's Guide to the Brain,* New York, Pantheon, 1998

Panksepp, J. *Affective Neuroscience: The Foundations of Human and Animal Emotions,* New York, Oxford University Press, 1998

ADHD

Hallowell, E. M. and Ratey, J. J. *Driven to Distraction,* New York, Pantheon, 1994

Hallowell, E. M. and Ratey, J. J. *Answers to Distraction,* New York, Pantheon, 1995

Hartmann, T. *Attention Deficit Disorder: A Different Perception,* Novato, Underwood-Miller, 1993

Hartmann, T. and Bowman, J. *Think Fast: the ADD Experience,* Grass Valley, Underwood, 1996

Hartmann, T. *ADD Success Stories: A Guide to Fulfillment for Families with Attention Deficit Disorder,* Grass Valley, Underwood, 1995

Dynamics, Oppositional Children

Bustamante, E. *Parenting the AD/HD Child: A New Approach,* Springfield, Whitcomb, 1997

Exercise

Kirkpatrick, B. and Birnbaum, B. H. *Lessons From The Heart: Individualizing Physical Education With Heart Rate Monitors,* Champaigne, Human Kinetics, 1997

Edwards, S. *The Heart Rate Monitor Book,* Woodbury, Polar Electro Oy, 1993

Sleamaker, R. *Serious Training for Serious Athletes,* Champaign, Leisure, 1989

Crawling Exercises for ADHD

Cook, P., O'Dell, N., *Stopping Hyperactivity, a new solution,* Avery, 1997.

Gold, S. J., *If Kids Just Came with Instruction Sheets!,* Eugene, Fern Ridge, 1997

Index

Jokyl, E. 21
Journal 64-66, 108-116
Junger, S. 9, 117

Marathon mind 10, 30
Medication, pros/cons 13, 14
Medication withdrawal 16
Mind/body connection, 90
Motivation 51, 52
Motivational process 77-78
Motivational techniques, 81-85

Neurochemicals, 33-35
Novelty seeking 53-54

Opposition 63
Optimal stimulation 21-22, 24-26, 32
Optimism 114
Over-training 120-122, 124
Outward Bound 9

Panksepp, J. 10, 31-32, 59-60
Parental roles 60-63
Physician 16, 18, 20, 99, 118-119
Placebo effect 40, 41
Play 31, 32
Positive Addiction 28, 41
Proprioceptive feedback 22
Psychological intensity, 107
Psychostimulants 36

Ratey, J. 31, 42
Reward 28, 29, 32-33, 36
Rickshas 62
Ritalin 9
Ritalin, effects on play 10
Rough housing 59-60
Runner's high 27-28, 37

Safety 117-125
    Sport-specific 118, 123-124

Scott, T. 48, 61
Self concept 114
Self esteem, 28
Shipman, W. M. 5-8, 45-46, 61
St. John's Anglican Boarding
    School 9-10, 23, 46, 60, 66
Stimulus deprivation 21, 22, 25
Stretching 120
Substance abuse 113

Walking 71-72
Warm-up 120
Weights 47

For information about Upper Access Books, contact:

Upper Access, Inc., Book Publishers
PO Box 457 • 87 Upper Access Road
Hinesburg, VT 05461
802/482-2988
Toll-Free Phone for Orders Only: 1-800-310-8320
E-mail *info@upperaccess.com* • Web *www.upperaccess.com*

About the Author . . .

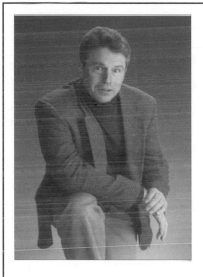

Stephen C. Putnam holds an
M.Ed. degree in Guidance and
Psychological Services from
Springfield College. As an adult
marathon paddler, Steve's life was
changed by the magic of exercise.
Among other things, he learned
that tranquility is not just a concept. Canoe racing became a family activity. At different times,
paddling allowed his son, Adam,
and daughter, Heather, to take
charge as stern paddlers. The fun provided the initial research and
insight that nature might supply the Ritalin. As it turned out,
dopamine deprivation is correctable.